SINUS SURVIVAL

SINUS SURVIVAL

THE HOLISTIC MEDICAL TREATMENT FOR ALLERGIES, ASTHMA, BRONCHITIS, COLDS, AND SINUSITIS

Third Edition, Revised and Expanded

ROBERT S. IVKER, D.O.

President-Elect, American Holistic Medical Association

Foreword by Robert A. Anderson, M.D.

A Jeremy P. Tarcher/Putnam Book
Published by G. P. Putnam's Sons
NEW YORK

Most Tarcher/Putnam books are available at special quantity discounts for bulk purchases for sales promotions, premiums, fund-raising, and educational needs. Special books or book excerpts also can be created to fit specific needs.
For details, write or telephone Special Markets, The Putnam Publishing Group, 200 Madison Avenue, New York, NY 10016; (212) 951-8891.

A Jeremy P. Tarcher/Putnam Book
Published by G. P. Putnam's Sons
Publishers Since 1838
200 Madison Avenue
New York, NY 10016
http://www.putnam.com/putnam

The author wishes to thank the following for permission to reprint their material in this book:
Photograph of steam inhaler courtesy of Bernhard Industries, Inc.; photograph of CAT scan courtesy of Bruce W. Jafek, M.D., F.A.C.S.; anatomical illustrations and exercise diagrams by Eileen Rudnick; Candida score sheet from The Yeast Connection and the Woman by William G. Crook, M.D., Professional Books, Jackson, Tennessee, 1995, reprinted by permission of William G. Crook, M.D., and Professional Books. Excerpts from Optimal Wellness: Where Mainstream and Alternative Medicine Meet by Ralph Golan, M.D., New York, Ballantine Books, 1995, reprinted by permission of Ralph Golan, M.D.

Charts pages 176–84 © 1995 by Robert S. Ivker

Library of Congress Cataloging-in-Publication Data

Ivker, Robert S.
   Sinus survival : the holistic medical treatment for allergies, asthma, bronchitis, colds, and sinusitis / by Robert S. Ivker ; foreword by Robert A. Anderson.—3rd ed., rev. and expanded.
      p. cm.
   Includes bibliographical references and index.
   ISBN 0-87477-807-7
   1. Sinusitis—Popular works. 2. Cold (Disease)—Popular works.
3. Respiratory allergy—Popular works. 4. Bronchitis—Popular works. I. Title.
RF425.I84   1995
616.2—dc20   95-17371 CIP

Book design by Susan Hood
Cover design by Tanya Maiboroda
Cover photograph of air pollution © Telegraph Colour Library/FPG
Cover photograph of ripening barley © David Woodfall/Tony Stone Images
Photograph of author by Nancy Zorensky

Printed in the United States of America

20 19 18 17

This book is printed on acid-free paper. ∞

To my daughters, Julie and Carin, for teaching me to be a better player in the game of life and for creating a wealth of opportunities for taking life much less seriously.

CONTENTS

Contents

ACKNOWLEDGMENTS

This third edition of *Sinus Survival* was edited by Laura Golden Bellotti, and I am most grateful to her for the additions and revisions that she so gracefully made. The majority of the text, originally and masterfully edited by Mary Ellen Strote, has remained unchanged.

The physicians who have helped me in creating the new material in this book are Bob Anderson, Sylvia Flesner, Ralph Golan, Milton Ivker, Bruce Jafek, George Kitchie, Ann McCombs, Steve Morris, and Todd Nelson. Thank you for your time and valuable input. Rex Coppom and Carl Grimes contributed to the additions and revisions in Chapter 7.

To the many patients who had been ill for so long with candida, I am deeply indebted. Your suffering and subsequent commitment and recovery have taught me more than I could have ever learned in the course of formal medical training. You have made a profound contribution to the Sinus Survival Program, one that will ultimately benefit many others who are similarly afflicted. I'd like to specifically acknowledge George Klabin, Patti Ludlam, Claude Selitrennikoff, John Snider, and Claire Zimmerman for your help with the "Candida" chapter.

Thanks also to the hundreds of patients, letter writers, and readers who responded to the Sinus Survival Questionnaire. Much of the information that you've provided me is included in this book.

A special thanks to Jeremy Tarcher—a publisher with vision.

Acknowledgments

The courage you've displayed in maintaining your commitment to holistic health, and the success you've enjoyed as a result, should serve as an inspiration to the entire publishing industry. Thanks for the opportunity you've afforded me, and for helping to enhance the quality of life for millions, with a multitude of your paradigm-shifting books.

Most of all, I'd like to thank my wife, Harriet, for contributing a great deal to the "Social Health" and "Candida" chapters and for your patience, understanding, and support in taking care of the rest of my life while I was so totally immersed in this project. Your love has played a major role in my own "sinus survival."

FOREWORD

Many authorities past and present have debated the nature of disease. In the 1860s Louis Pasteur promoted the concept of microorganisms—viruses, bacteria—as the cause of disease. An arch-rival, Claude Bernard, argued that the "milieu interieur" was most important. A susceptible "constitution," he said, was the essence of disease. In a modern era, we would rephrase his argument: *Weakening of the immune system makes human beings susceptible to the ravages of invaders*—microorganisms, toxins, and allergenic substances. Conventional medicine is focused on the antibiotic actions of drugs. Beyond this approach, holistic medicine in addition emphasizes prevention, health promotion, and enhancement of the immune and antioxidant defenses of the body. The possibility and validity of improving the function of the immune system is not accepted by most authorities today.

Any new concept appearing in the fabric of our culture is always met with skepticism and the subtle problem of "institutional delay." The first known paper regarding scurvy and citrus fruit appeared in a publication of the London Medical Society in 1796. The British navy did not adopt a mandatory policy requiring one piece of citrus fruit a day for maritime and navy seamen until after 1900, a delay of 108 years.

The earliest paper that definitively pointed out the essential nature of magnesium in heart disease dates from 1956. Yet major cardiology journals did not commonly discuss magnesium's importance in cardiac disease until the late 1980s. Whenever evolutionary or revolutionary concepts reshape a new paradigm, we fall heir to insidious institutional delay.

A foremost question, then, during times of rapid cultural change, is where to look for credible information and to be able to dissect out the truth as it is understood at the moment.

Fortunately for the human species, the result of thought allows us to assess ourselves as we currently understand ourselves to be, pondering whether the system of which we are a part is serving us well. By analogy, if we have traditionally purchased goods and services from a particular dealer or practitioner, and we sense we are not doing well, we give ourselves permission to change and seek new sources for assistance. If our health is deteriorating, we may then choose to look for alternatives, learn about new possibilities, and make interim judgments as we proceed.

Again, by analogy, when we find a new store that merchandises goods that manifest for us utility, quality, and longevity, we tend to return to that store for more products. We also get a sense of how we're doing when we use a new concept for a time—such as physical activity, meditation, or the intentional systematic use of the imagination. In other words, simply trying it out. And what about others? Are those folks who seem to be doing the best in society using the new concept?

Dr. Ivker emphasizes the concept of unconditional love as a powerful life medicine. The attitude of unconditional love is integral to concepts of managing the ubiquitous "stress" in the lives of all of us, without succumbing to its potential devastating effects. And when we evaluate the status of those embracing unconditional love as their most important medicine, we can judge its value for us. And, often, we see these self-actualized individuals joyfully contributing to life well into their ninth and tenth decades.

There is a time-tested principle of looking at the health professional and asking: Is the message "Do as I do," or "Do as I say"? At a recent American Heart Association annual meeting, one of the researchers presented a paper reporting a significant reduction in heart disease in a group of subjects who took supplements of vitamin E compared to those who did not. Asked afterward if he took vitamin E supplements personally, he emphatically answered, yes, he did. When asked if he recommended it for patients he stated, "No. Until we have absolute, incontrovertible, irrevocable proof that it works, I can't recommend it." "Do as I say" meant "don't take vitamin E supplements."

Medical research monies in Western culture are unfortunately almost exclusively spent investigating disease in the ill portion of the population. And this is important. We should, however, spend equivalent amounts researching the healthy and the well, especially the happy, productive, alert, vital seniors in their eighties and nineties. How did they do it? We know heredity contributes to longevity and extended quality of life, but lifestyle makes quintessential contributions as well. The commitment, control, and challenge to which Kobasa refers is the essence of hardiness. How did these hardy seniors structure their lives to balance their nutrition, exercise, environmental concerns, thinking, beliefs, social interactions, and challenge to be able to continue contributing and serving society in their eighties and nineties?

The new paradigm moves from the debate about the true nature of disease to a debate about the true nature of health. The view that Dr. Ivker brings into focus is integrally related to the nature of health. What does it mean to be well, whole, healed, joyful, productive, and having reverence for life? What is the nature of the immune system poised to handle the stresses of life, whether they be environmental, toxic, infectious, or allergenic in nature? The answers to these questions will gradually be surfacing in the next several years. The answers form the matrix of the new paradigm, and Rob Ivker is a leader in the defining and grounding of its principles.

The journey to finding the answers will be exciting!

—ROBERT A. ANDERSON, M.D.

Robert A. Anderson, author of Wellness Medicine *and* Stress Power!, *is a former clinical assistant professor in the Department of Family Medicine at the University of Washington School of Medicine. He is also a cofounder and past president of the American Holistic Medical Association.*

PREFACE

In the seven years since the first edition of *Sinus Survival* was written and published (November 1988), we have witnessed the emergence of America's first environmental epidemic—sinusitis. It remains our most common chronic or "incurable" disease, afflicting one out of every seven people in the United States. But even more startling is the fact that acute sinusitis (sinus infection) may have already replaced the common cold as our most frequent illness. In a research study performed at the University of Virginia in 1993, students who thought they had a *cold* were evaluated with CT scans—the most diagnostic test for sinusitis. The scans revealed that 87 percent did not have a simple cold, but in fact had a *sinus infection*!

The majority of the public and the medical community are still largely unaware of the extent to which this debilitating and insidious problem is adversely affecting us. The pharmaceutical and advertising companies, however, are very clearly "tuned in" to the magnitude of the epidemic. From November 1993 through March 1994, the most often-aired commercials on ABC, CBS, and NBC-TV were for cold and sinus remedies. The combined revenue from these ads exceeded $600 million! During this same time frame, sinus problems were highlighted on both NBC and ABC no fewer than eleven times during the network news with Tom Brokaw and Peter Jennings. What a tremendous amount of attention and money for a problem that few people had even heard of ten years ago. The National Center for Health Statistics has confirmed that the plague of sinus disease is growing. Chronic sinusitis remains America's most common chronic or "incurable" ailment, while three other respiratory conditions are also among the ten most common chronic diseases —allergies (number 5), chronic bronchitis (number 8), and asthma (number 9). Together, these four respiratory diseases afflict more than 92 million people, about 35 percent of our population.

Since the first edition was published, we have also seen significant changes in both causes and treatment of chronic sinusitis. Along with a myriad of new antibiotics, endoscopic sinus surgery has seen a meteoric rise. When conventional sinus treatments fail, most of these "treatment-failures" eventually find themselves being referred to a sinus specialist—an ear, nose, and throat surgeon. Since the medical treatment didn't work, these physicians usually waste little time in recommending surgery as their solution. In 1995 the number of these surgeries will exceed 500,000, costing our health care system nearly *$5 billion!* If it cured the problem, we might be able to justify this prohibitive expense, but, unfortunately for most patients, sinus surgery has become a high-tech and expensive form of treating symptoms. Ironically, the conventional medical treatment for acute sinusitis —powerful broad-spectrum antibiotics—has been partially responsible for creating the sinus crisis. More people are becoming resistant to the antibiotics, there is mounting evidence that antibiotics may actually be weakening our immune system, and millions of others are developing a yeast overgrowth called candidiasis as a result of taking antibiotics. Candidiasis often causes greater illness than chronic sinusitis alone. During the past decade, the overgrowth of *Candida albicans,* a yeast organism normally found in the bowel, may have become an even more pervasive epidemic than sinusitis. It can wreak havoc throughout the bodies of those suffering from it, and especially their sinuses.

This condition, candidiasis, is currently the primary cause of disease in almost 90 percent of my patients with type 1 chronic sinusitis. Yet seven years ago I wasn't even aware of its existence. Although it is difficult to treat, I have learned a great deal about this condition. The new chapter "Candida" represents the greatest amount of new material in this book.

As a "last-resort" doctor, I routinely work with the most challenging cases of sinusitis. I see many people who have had multiple surgical procedures before coming to see me. One woman actually had fourteen sinus surgeries. At this point in its evolution, the Sinus Survival Program described in this book is guaranteed to make a profound difference in the health status of anyone willing to make the commitment to him or herself. As I will relate in greater detail in the final chapters, while the majority of my patients have cured their chronic sinusitis, many of them have also transformed their lives in the process.

As health care reform seeks to control spiraling costs, there is a growing sense of urgency to develop less expensive treatments for chronic disease, and a corresponding interest in preventive medicine. The National Institutes of Health (NIH) opened the Office of Alternative Medicine in 1992 to evaluate the therapeutic value and cost-effectiveness of "alternative" therapies. The study of the Sinus Survival Program was denied funding by this office because it was deemed not "alternative" enough (since drugs and surgery could still be used although very infrequently), and not focused on a single therapeutic modality. I explained that this program is "holistic medicine," and as such it treats body, mind, and spirit with a wide variety of safe, gentle, and inexpensive *complementary* therapies. Although my argument was for naught, many thousands of sinus sufferers, both patients and readers alike, can now attest to both the cost savings and their condition of well-being.

Even the medical establishment has taken notice. Thanks to the courage and foresight of Bruce Jafek, M.D., professor and chairman of the Department of Otolaryngology (ear, nose, and throat) at the University of Colorado School of Medicine, I was appointed clinical instructor in his department in 1994. It is most unusual for a family physician to be given such an appointment, let alone one who practices holistic medicine. In collaboration with Dr. Jafek, we have created the Nasal and Sinus Diseases Center at the University of Colorado Health Sciences Center. One of Dr. Jafek's primary goals in the establishment of this sinus center is to scientifically study the effectiveness of the Sinus Survival Program and ultimately make it a much more available option to sinus patients through ENT physicians.

Sinus Survival has always been a self-help guide. In preparing for this third edition, I mailed nearly two thousand questionnaires to patients whom I've personally worked with on the Sinus Survival Program and readers of the book whom I've never met. From the hundreds of questionnaire responses and letters I've received from readers, in addition to the experience I've gained from working with very sick patients, I've attempted to make this book the most user-friendly edition yet. In the chapter entitled "The Top 10," I have answered the ten questions most frequently asked by patients, readers, and letter writers. There is also a great deal of new information about asthma, allergies, bronchitis, antibiotics, holistic and osteopathic medicine, as well as updated material on treating your environment. I've included new diagrams and charts to make it easier to learn how to both diagnose and treat your condition. I've made it possible for you to obtain many of the products that are mentioned throughout the text by including a "Product Index" at the end of the book. Every chapter contains something that's new.

It has been almost three and a half years since I wrote the second edition. We live in a very rapidly changing world, one in which our environment is being destroyed at an astounding rate. We, as a global community, must realize that as we devastate our natural world, especially the air we breathe, we may be threatening our own survival. Sinusitis could be just the tip of the iceberg. As we look toward the twenty-first century, health care reform will increasingly push each of us to take more responsibility for our own health. Making ourselves healthier can be an exciting and enlivening process, but it entails much more than a scientific quick fix. It becomes a highly personalized labor of love. Let *Sinus Survival,* together with your ailing sinuses and your compassionate heart, become your guide on this healing journey!

ROB IVKER
February 1995

INTRODUCTION

In my medical career I have been responsible for the care of more than 20,000 patients with sinus problems. From 1977 to 1987, I worked hard to cure my own sinus condition (more about that later) and with my patients to dispel the belief that I and they would have to live indefinitely with the unpleasantness of sinusitis—despite the fact that conventional methods for treating it were becoming increasingly less effective.

Throughout my personal ten-year odyssey, I experimented with a myriad of therapeutic modalities, innovative techniques, and folk remedies. Most of my effort was focused on medical treatments, and those that were effective are all found in this book. This approach improved my sinuses; however, it was not until my healing journey took me into the exciting new frontier of holistic medicine that I achieved a cure. I have been free of chronic sinusitis for almost eight years. Since publication of the original edition of *Sinus Survival*, I have treated even more challenging sinus patients than I had seen before. They, too, experienced remarkable results. Through working with them, I have been able to refine some of the material from that first edition.

My need to practice "sinus survival" began in 1975 with my first sinus infection. I had suffered with seasonal allergies (also called hay fever) throughout most of my childhood, but this was something very different. Over the next three years, I had several more infections and finally developed chronic sinusitis. "Normal" for me now meant a stuffy head, frequent sinus headaches, and a lot of mucus drainage down the back of my throat. I consulted an ear, nose, and throat (ENT) specialist, who told me that there was no cure and that I would have to learn to live with it. I was stunned.

This young physician, who idealistically believed in the healing power of medical science, had just been given a strong dose of reality. The specialist's prognosis was a rude reminder that although modern medicine saves many lives and performs daily miracles, doctors are able to cure only about 25 percent of the ailments they treat. Chronic sinusitis is not among that select group. Although I had hardly been handed a death sentence, sinus disease was already having a profoundly negative impact on the quality of my life.

Ironically, it was to enhance my quality of life that I had come to Denver, Colorado, from Philadelphia in 1972. I entered a family practice residency training program, where I was taught that it was part of a family doctor's responsibility to teach patients about preventive medicine; in other words, how to stay well.

During my three years as a resident at Mercy Medical Center, I felt exhilarated whenever I caught a glimpse of the magnificent Rocky Mountains on the western edge of the city. With increasing frequency, however, that vista was obstructed with what later came to be known as "the brown cloud." Air pollution was quickly becoming a problem that Denver could no longer ignore.

After completing my residency, I took my family and newly developed sinus condition to the outskirts of the city, where I began a solo family practice. Being something of an amateur statistician, I kept track of the diagnoses of all of my patients. Through the mid- to late 1970s, acute sinusitis (sinus infection) was usually fourteenth or fifteenth on my list of the top twenty diagnoses. By 1982 it had become number one, and it has headed my list ever since. While compiling data from other family practices and residencies for a medical conference I was organizing, I found that my observation correlated with those of family doctors nationwide. Sinusitis was near the top of every list of the most common ailments being treated by family physicians. In the summer of 1981, the National Center for Health Statistics reported that chronic sinusitis had overtaken arthritis as the most common chronic disease in the United States.

I asked myself, Why this sudden epidemic of sinus disease? The answer came from above (the toxic cloud hovering over the city like a suffocating blanket) and from within (increasingly polluted indoor environments). There was no escape. Residents of the Mile-High City are not alone in their suffering: Almost every major urban center in the world is plagued with air pollution.

According to the Environmental Protection Agency (EPA), more than 150 million Americans—60 percent of the population —live in areas in which the air is hazardous to their health. But what is actually happening to us as a result of breathing this filthy air? That question has still not been addressed by any governmental agency. Part of my purpose in writing this book has been to offer my own theory about the devastating impact air pollution is having on human beings. I have included a section on indoor air pollution, a subject the EPA is now addressing as it identifies the multitude of pollutants found in our homes and workplaces.

Although it has not yet been conclusively proven in a laboratory, the hypothesis of an air pollution–sinus disease connection will certainly withstand scientific scrutiny. A primary function of the sinuses is to filter the air we breathe. We need only look at what we are breathing to appreciate that our sinuses are, at the very least, having to work much harder than they used to. After this book was first published late in 1988, I was invited to speak to the scientists at the Air Pollution Health Effects Laboratory at the University of California at Irvine. The director of the lab, Dr. Robert F. Phalen, has said, "There is scientific evidence relating air pollution to significant epithelial cell damage in the nasal cavity of the rat." This is solid support for the pollution–sinus disease link.

Sales of this book in bookstores and in physicians' offices have shown an interesting pattern. Sales have been highest in the cities and states the EPA has identified as having the dirtiest air: Los Angeles, Denver, New York, Ohio, Texas, Pennsylvania, Michigan, Illinois, and Tennessee. This evidence might not be scientific, but it surely scores some circumstantial points in support of my theory.

Sinus disease is difficult to identify for both doctor and patient. Most people with a sinus infection believe they have "a cold that just won't quit." In this book I offer a clinical description of both acute and chronic sinusitis, along with the other common respiratory ailments—allergic rhinitis, asthma, and acute and chronic bronchitis.

Using this book, you will be able to diagnose, treat, prevent, and—if you choose to make that level of commitment—cure yourself of the affliction of sinus and respiratory disease. This is a condition that easily lends itself to self-healing. Those free of sinus problems will learn the potential hazards of breathing polluted air and what they can do to protect themselves through the practice of preventive medicine. *Sinus Survival* provides a practical plan for living a full and healthy lifestyle in an increasingly unhealthy environment.

This book offers you many avenues of possible relief from sinus and respiratory disease. They all work. You will find many treatment options that offer rapid improvement of symptoms, and you will be given the opportunity to confront causes and take increased responsibility not only for the condition of your sinuses and lungs but also for your overall state of health. The holistic methods take longer to implement and they require more effort, but the improvement in your sinuses and general health will be far greater. The holistic program is a personalized approach to health based on learning to love yourself in each aspect of your life—environmental, physical, mental, emotional, spiritual, and social. Loving yourself is not a selfish indulgence, but rather a discovery, an appreciation, and an acceptance of the unique individual that you are. Through this work you will learn what feels good to you, how to provide it for yourself, and how to give more to others. You will experience a greater degree of health and vitality than you have ever had before.

Part I

AN INTRODUCTION TO SINUS AND RESPIRATORY DISEASE

Chapter 1

WHAT ARE SINUSES?

M ost people probably assume that the word *sinus* means "nose." They would be close, both anatomically and physiologically, but although the nose and sinuses are connected, they are separate parts of the body. The sinuses are air-filled cavities located behind and around the nose and eyes. In anatomy texts they are called air sinuses or paranasal sinuses. There are usually four sets, roughly divided in half for each side of the head. The halves can be asymmetrical in size and shape.

The sinuses are identified as frontal, maxillary, sphenoid, and ethmoid (Figure 1-1). The frontal sinuses lie above the eyes, just above the nose and behind the forehead. The maxillaries, the largest of the sinuses, are pyramid-shaped cavities located inside each cheekbone. The ethmoids, multicompartmental sinuses behind the maxillaries and between the bony orbits of the eyes, are complex labyrinths of small air pockets. The sphenoids are situated deep in the skull behind the nose, slightly below the ethmoids. The ethmoidal, sphenoidal, and maxillary sinuses are all present at birth, although the latter do not reach full development until a person is sixteen to twenty-one years of age. The frontal sinuses are not present until the age of eight.

To make mucus drainage and air exchange possible, each sinus is connected to the nasal passage by a thin duct about the size of pencil lead. The openings of the ducts are called ostia, and they

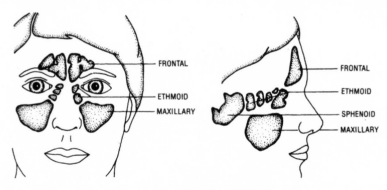

FIGURE 1-1. *Location of Sinuses*

average about two millimeters in diameter. The ducts of the maxillaries are located at the top of the sinus, making drainage difficult and blockage easy. A series of small ducts in the nasal wall drain the ethmoid sinuses; these openings are also easily blocked. Although most of the human body seems to have been created perfectly, the maxillary sinuses are a distinct exception. They appear to be better suited to four-legged animals, particularly with regard to the position of the ostia. As upright posture evolved, ease of sinus drainage diminished.

One kind of tissue, the respiratory epithelium, lines the sinuses, the nose, and the lungs. All three are part of the respiratory tract (Figure 1-2), which performs the essential function of breathing. The outermost part of the epithelium is called the mucosa. This is a continuous mucous membrane lining the sinuses, ducts, and nasal passages. Therefore, anything that causes a swelling in the nose can similarly affect the sinuses. On the surface of this membrane are cilia, microscopic hairlike filaments that maintain a constant sweeping motion to remove the watery discharge called mucus (Figure 1-3).

The mucous membrane and its cilia provide a good defensive mechanism against infections. The entire mucus covering of the maxillary sinus, for example, is normally cleared every ten minutes. The mucous membrane lining the entire respiratory tract

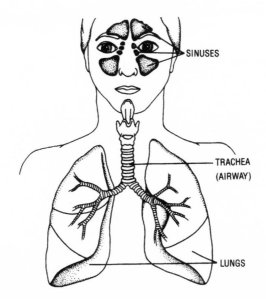

FIGURE 1-2. *The Respiratory Tract*

produces between a pint and a quart of mucus daily. The mucus traps particles that enter the nasal passage, and the cilia sweep them toward the back of the nose, after which they are swallowed and broken down by stomach acids.

No one has definitively established the exact function of the sinuses, although there is agreement that they lighten the weight of the skull. By virtue of the sinuses' location and structure and the microanatomy and function of the mucous membrane, most physiologists would agree with the following conclusions.

The sinuses, along with the nose, as the upper part of the respiratory tract, serve as the body's chief protector of the lungs. They do this by acting as a *filter,* defending against bacteria and viruses, dirt and dust particles, pollen, and anything airborne that would harm the lungs; as a *humidifier,* by moistening dry air that would irritate the lungs; and as a *temperature regulator,* by cooling excessively hot air and warming extremely cold air that would shock the lungs. Humans inhale about 23,000 times a day, mov-

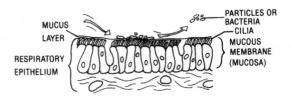

FIGURE 1-3. *The Sinus Lining, Healthy*

ing the equivalent of about two gallons of air per minute—almost 3,000 gallons per day. The nose and sinuses are always at work, shielding the lungs from harm. Our lungs are the vehicle through which our bodies obtain oxygen, which is vital to life itself.

The sinuses are the lungs' leading defenders against injury and illness, but their importance has been neglected by both doctors and patients. Think about a quarterback on the football field whose offensive line is weak and beginning to break down. He might not be killed, literally, but what about his health and his ability to perform optimally? Our nose and sinuses are being assaulted and are beginning to deteriorate. The condition of our lungs is already being affected, and ultimately the health of our bodies is at stake. Let us see how we might help to create optimum health by reinforcing our first line of defense, the sinuses.

Chapter 2

WHAT MAKES SINUSES SICK?

Today more than one out of every seven Americans (38 million people) is a sinus sufferer. Sinus disease has become an epidemic. Although some factors are more critical than others, the cause of any illness is always multifaceted. The multiple causes of this epidemic will be discussed in this chapter. They have the potential to affect adversely even the healthiest sinus. However, a person who has had previous sinus problems or whose sinuses have been weakened for any of the reasons mentioned here is already at high risk for developing sinusitis. The following agents are involved: the common cold, cigarettes and other sources of smoke, air pollution, dry air, cold air, fumes, allergies, occupational hazards, dental problems, immunodeficiency, malformations, and emotional stress.

THE COMMON COLD

The story of what has become a lifetime of sinus problems usually began with the common cold. Normally, air and mucus flow freely through the ducts connecting the nose and sinuses. Trouble starts when the system becomes obstructed, usually by a cold. The nasal mucous membrane becomes inflamed and swollen and the cold virus inactivates the cilia of the nasal membrane, causing

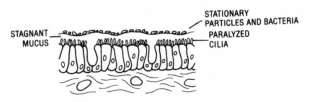

FIGURE 2-1. *The Sinus Lining, Sinusitis*

the mucus in the nose to stagnate rather than flow (Figure 2-1). As a result, the mucus being produced in the sinuses cannot drain properly, and the sinuses become a breeding ground for bacteria. This pooling of stagnant mucus can easily result in a sinus infection, especially in individuals who have had previous infections.

Through the early and mid–1970s, I treated many patients who had nothing more than a bad cold. By the late seventies, and certainly by the early eighties, patients with the common cold became less frequent visitors to my office. They were being replaced by patients who greeted me with complaints such as, "Doctor, I've had this cold for the past two weeks now" (or three weeks, or several months, or in a few cases, a year or more). These people almost always had sinusitis, and not until they had completed a course of antibiotics were they able to rid themselves of their "cold." It also became quite apparent that those who had never before had a sinus infection were now frequently returning with the same problem.

In the Preface I referred to landmark research performed in 1993 by Dr. Jack Gwaltney at the University of Virginia at Charlottesville. He studied college students and employees who thought they had the common cold. Following CT or "cat" scans, the most definitive diagnostic test to evaluate sinuses, 87 percent of these people were found to have sinus infections. What I began observing in my family practice more than fifteen years ago had now been scientifically documented—the vast majority of people who think they have a simple cold actually have a sinus infection, called acute sinusitis, as an integral part of the cold. After a first bout with sinusitis, the mucous membrane, especially its cilia, is left in a somewhat damaged and weakened state. For many, the membrane never completely recovers, especially in an environment that is harsh on the sinuses. What I was seeing, increasingly, was that one or two "bad colds" could result in a permanently weak sinus. This impaired sinus then becomes much more susceptible to additional infections, whether from a cold or any of the other risk factors that follow.

CIGARETTES AND OTHER SOURCES OF SMOKE

Whenever a patient with a sinus infection returned to my office after completing a two-week, or longer, course of antibiotics and complained, "Doctor, I'm not any better," my first response was always a question: "Have you been smoking?" The patient often answered yes. It is extremely difficult to have healthy sinuses if you smoke cigarettes. Nicotine paralyzes the cilia. I would be hard pressed to name anything more harmful to the body's air filter than smoke of any kind. Cigarette smoke is most often involved, but cigar, pipe, campfire, and cooking smoke are also frequent villains. Marijuana and cocaine (whether smoked or snorted) are also quite harmful to the nasal mucous membrane.

If you are curious about what smoke does to the sinuses, take a look at the accumulation of tar and smoke particles that discolor a used cigarette filter, turning it brown or black. This will give you some idea of what is happening not only to the sinuses, but also to the lungs. At the tissue level, smoke causes irritation of the mucous membrane. The weaker the sinus, usually one that has been infected previously, the greater the level of irritation. The greater the irritation, the more inflamed the mucous membrane becomes. Inflammation of the mucous membrane results in swelling, increased mucus secretion, and damage to the cilia. This swelling may obstruct the sinuses, producing a condition very similar to that created by the common cold.

When fluids or secretions are unable to drain normally, the

potential for infection is high. This principle holds true for almost any part of the human body, whether it is the bladder, bowel, lung, kidney, or middle ear space. The theory that smoking can cause sinus infections has not yet been proven. It is currently beyond the scope of science to observe what is happening to the mucous membrane in someone's sinus as it is being suffocated with smoke. However, as with the speculation on the function of the sinuses, this theory, too, has strong support among most physicians.

Those of you who are sinus sufferers but do not smoke are not necessarily immune to the problems caused by cigarette and other types of smoke. Recent studies have shown that nonsmokers who live or work with smokers are also adversely affected. New laws that prohibit cigarette smoking in public places are helping, but we have a long way to go.

In 1992, a Harvard research team reported the first direct medical evidence that secondhand smoke can damage the lungs of nonsmokers. The study reported that secondhand smoke:

- kills at least 4,000 people annually from lung cancer;
- increases the risk of respiratory infections in children;
- aggravates the symptoms of asthma in children.

The American Heart Association estimates that, in addition to its effects on lungs, secondhand smoke could be a contributing factor in the heart-disease deaths of 40,000 nonsmoking Americans every year. The association also estimates that 50 million nonsmoking adults over the age of thirty-five are exposed to secondhand smoke and about 50 percent of all American children live in families with one or more smokers.

As yet, there is no direct scientific data on what secondhand smoke is doing to our nose and sinuses. But with this recent evidence documenting its devastating effects on our lungs and hearts, it's obviously not too speculative to assume that secondhand smoke is also causing significant damage to the body's air filter.

AIR POLLUTION: OUTDOOR

I was struck by a comment made several years ago by one of the Apollo astronauts. He said that the most disturbing part of his flight was seeing a grayish haze over almost every land mass on earth. What was this ugly blanket covering our beautiful planet?

Having lived in Denver, I had a good clue. The Mile-High City, one of this country's most polluted metropolitan areas, is often covered by a thick, brownish-gray pall of smog, known locally as the brown cloud. Most cities in the world are similarly afflicted, but especially those situated in valleys where temperature inversions are frequent; in cities where diesel fuel is used extensively, especially in Europe; in heavily industrialized regions; and in most areas where there are coal-fired power plants. Almost every country in the world is now familiar with this rapidly growing dilemma; it has reached such immense proportions that it is visible from space. The question is, what is this filthy air doing to the human beings who created the problem?

In Denver, the incidence of acute sinusitis has risen dramatically since the early 1970s. Since 1982, it has consistently been the most common illness in my medical practice. Is it only a coincidence that during the same period of time air pollution has undergone a similar meteoric rise? In Denver, air pollution is most acute from mid-November to mid-January, when temperature inversions—warm air aloft trapping cold air and pollutants near the ground—are most common. This also happens to be the time of year when Denver's doctors see the greatest number of sinus infections. Many people who work in the center of the city or in other highly polluted areas are aware of the connection between their sinus congestion and sinus headaches on days with particularly bad air quality.

There is scientific evidence to implicate carbon monoxide as the most dangerous element of air pollution. Why? Because, in high enough concentrations, it is capable of killing people with weak hearts and lungs. It is also the component of air pollution most often measured, and we know that about 25 percent of it comes from vehicle emissions.

According to the EPA's 1993 National Air Quality and Emissions Trends Report, the metropolitan areas with the highest eight-hour concentration of carbon monoxide in that year were:

1. Los Angeles–Long Beach, CA
2. Spokane, WA
3. El Paso, TX
4. (tie) Denver, CO
   Anchorage, AK
   Las Vegas, NV-AZ
   Provo–Orem, UT
5. (tie) Steubenville–Weirton, OH
   Albuquerque, NM
   Phoenix–Mesa, AZ
   Memphis, TN-AR-MS
   Las Cruces, NM
   Sacramento, CA
   Baton Rouge, LA

All of these cities met or exceeded the federal limit of carbon monoxide for eight hours. But carbon monoxide is an odorless and colorless gas. What is that stuff that we can see—the brown cloud—and what is it doing to our sinuses when we breathe it?

Visible pollution consists primarily of the following elements: particulates, oxides of sulfur, oxides of nitrogen, hydrocarbons, and ozone. Particulates are tiny particles of dust, sand, cinders, soot, smoke, and liquid droplets found in the atmosphere. They come from a variety of sources, including roads, farm fields, construction sites, factories, power plants, fireplaces, wood-burning stoves, windblown dust, and diesel and car exhaust. When inhaled, larger particles (those greater than 10 microns in diameter; a human hair is about 75 microns in diameter) are known to lodge in the nose and sinuses. After all, what is a filter for? While the large particles seem to have the greatest adverse impact on the nose and sinuses, those smaller than 10 microns are doing the most damage to the lungs.

In 1993, calculations emerging from studies at the Environmental Protection Agency and the Harvard School of Public Health estimate that 50,000 to 60,000 deaths a year are caused by particulate pollution. This number far surpasses that of any other pollutant and is one that rivals the death toll from some cancers. The most harmful particles are small—less than 10 microns in diameter—and are produced chiefly from industrial plants and to a lesser extent from the exhaust of diesel vehicles.

The federal government's current standard for these small particulates, called PM-10, doesn't consider air hazardous until it reaches 150 micrograms of these particles per cubic meter. Yet a recent study conducted in the Utah Valley found that hospital admissions for respiratory-related illnesses such as pneumonia and asthma jumped 50 to 90 percent during the times particulate pollution was above only 50 micrograms of breathable particles for each cubic meter of air. It may be time for the EPA to change the standard for particulates.

Although our nation spends about $35 billion a year on scrubbers, catalytic converters, and other air-pollution control efforts, only one-third of that money is aimed at removing particulates, and just a fraction of that goes toward the small PM-10 particles. Most regulatory efforts have been focused more on other types of pollutants, such as ozone and sulphur dioxide, that have been shown to damage health; it is uncertain whether they cause death. Aside from particulates, the EPA believes that, of all pollutants, indoor pollution, especially secondhand cigarette smoke, and radon cause the greatest health damage.

Scientists, unfortunately, are reluctant to establish conclusively a cause-and-effect relationship between particulates and respiratory disease until they have detailed biological studies of the effect of the PM-10 particles on the respiratory mucous membranes themselves. It's difficult to estimate how long that might take. Particulates, with their adverse health effects, however, have been around for a long time. Such pollution has been recorded as early as the seventeenth century in England. Today the effects may be more subtle but just as devastating. Deaths from particulates occur primarily among children with respiratory problems (mostly asthma), people of all ages with asthma, and the elderly with illnesses such as bronchitis, emphysema, and pneumonia. A comment from C. Arden Pope, Ph.D., one of the researchers in the Harvard particulate study (officially called the "Harvard Six Cities Study"), was most revealing. He said, "People who live in highly polluted cities die earlier. It's just that simple."

One of the largest studies of air quality and health ever carried out was published in the March 1995 issue of the *American Journal of Respiratory and Critical Care Medicine*. Performed by researchers from the Harvard School of Public Health and Brigham Young University, the study tracked the health records of 552,138 people in 151 cities between 1982 and 1989. The findings showed that fine particles, smaller than 2.5 microns, can increase the risk of death by 15 percent in cities with the dirtiest air, compared with the cleanest cities. This study bolsters the earlier Harvard study that showed particulates are costing tens of thousands of lives each year in the United States.

The act of breathing in those cities highest in particulates might be comparable to rubbing a piece of very fine sandpaper (particles larger than 10 microns constitute a coarser piece) against the delicate and sensitive mucous membranes of the entire respiratory tract, 23,000 times a day, day in and day out. The larger particulates, not usually measured by the EPA, take more of a toll on the "gatekeeper filter"—the nose and sinuses—while the smaller ones, less than 2.5 microns, are most devastating to the lungs.

According to the EPA's 1993 National Air Quality and Emissions Report, the metropolitan areas with the highest average particulate (PM-10) concentrations that year were, in descending order:

1. Riverside–San Bernardino, CA
2. Bakersfield, CA
3. (tie) Fresno, CA
   Visalia–Tulare–Porterville, CA

New Haven, Meriden, CT
4. Cleveland–Lorain–Elyria, OH
5. (tie) Chicago, IL
   Los Angeles–Long Beach, CA
   New York, NY
6. Spokane, WA
7. Reno, NV
8. (tie) Kansas City, MO-KS
   Las Vegas, NV-AZ
   Phoenix–Mesa, AZ
   St. Louis, MO
9. Merced, CA
10. (tie) Detroit, MI
    Rapid City, SD
    Denver, CO

Oxides of sulfur, especially sulfur dioxide (a colorless gas with a rotten-egg odor), are typically transformed into smaller, finer particulates, less than ten microns in diameter. Emitted mainly by coal- and oil-fired power plants, refineries, pulp and paper mills, and nonferrous smelters, they are a major contributor to acid rain, and are also filtered through the sinuses. Unfortunately, there is a price to be paid for protecting the lungs from this toxic substance. Sulfur oxide particles easily penetrate the mucosal lining. Studies have shown that they have an intensely irritating effect on the bronchial mucosa, resulting in damage to the cilia and initiation of bronchitis. If sulfur oxides can cause bronchitis in the lungs, would it be a farfetched assumption that they can also cause sinusitis?

According to the EPA's 1993 National Air Quality and Emissions Trends Report, the metropolitan areas with the highest amounts of sulfur dioxide were:

1. Steubenville–Weirton, OH-WV
2. Pittsburgh, PA
3. Billings, MT
4. Nashville, TN

5. Las Cruces, NM
6. Huntington–Ashland, WV-KY-OH
7. Youngstown–Warren, OH
8. Evansville–Henderson, IN-KY
9. St. Louis, MO
10. Cleveland–Lorain–Elyria, OH

Nitrogen oxides are the most obvious components of smog, providing color to the noxious cloud of air pollution. Their principal constituent is nitrogen dioxide, a yellowish-brown, highly reactive gas. Nitrogen oxides form when fuel is burned at high temperatures. The two major emission sources are internal combustion engines—motor vehicles and aircraft—and stationary fuel combustion sources such as electric utilities and industrial boilers. Like sulfur oxides, nitrogen oxides can irritate the lungs, causing ciliary paralysis, bronchitis, and pneumonia. They are also capable of impairing the body's immune defenses against bacterial and viral infection.

Los Angeles County is the only area in the country exceeding the federal nitrogen dioxide standard. The other cities that are highest in this pollutant are:

2. New York, NY
3. Riverside–San Bernardino, CA
4. Orange County, CA
5. Philadelphia, PA
6. Newark, NJ
7. Denver, CO
8. Boston, MA-NH
9. Baltimore, MD
10. Chicago, IL

Hydrocarbons are evaporated or incompletely burned organic compounds. The largest sources of hydrocarbons in the atmosphere include internal combustion engines; certain industrial processes, such as coke ovens in steel mills; and evaporation of liquids, such as gasoline in fuel transfers, and industrial and household solvents. Hydrocarbons are known to be highly irritating to the mucous membrane.

Prior to the recent findings about particulates, ozone was believed to be the most dangerous component of smog. It is produced when sunlight acts upon nitrogen oxides and hydrocarbons. The many sources of both of these substances have already been mentioned. Ozone in the lower, breathable part of the atmosphere (within 1,000 feet of the earth's surface) is harmful to human and animal health, crops, and forests. In the upper atmosphere, ozone is beneficial, absorbing the harmful rays (ultraviolet-B) of sunlight. The continuing depletion of the upper ozone layer has become a serious health concern. Unfortunately, harmful ozone in the lower air does not move up to replenish the deteriorating ozone layer in the higher reaches of our atmosphere.

Ozone in the lower atmosphere is one of our greatest environmental challenges. Few, if any, urban areas are free of it. Four broad geographic regions are seriously affected: Southern California (by far the worst), the Northeast (especially the New York City area), the Texas Gulf Coast, and the Chicago–Milwaukee area. Cities with the worst ozone pollution all exceeding federal standards, are:

1. Los Angeles–Long Beach, CA
2. Riverside–San Bernardino, CA
3. Houston, TX
4. Galveston–Texas City, TX
5. (tie) Orange County, CA
   Bridgeport, CT
6. (tie) Bakersfield, CA
   San Diego, CA
   Atlanta, GA
   Worcester, MA-CT
7. (tie) Hartford, CT
   Baltimore, MD
   Stamford–Norwalk, CT
   New Haven–Meriden, CT

Sacramento, CA
Visalia–Tulare–Potterville, CA

A growing body of scientific data indicates that ozone is a significant risk to human health, affecting not only those with impaired respiratory systems, such as asthmatics, but many with healthy lungs, both children and adults. Ozone can cause shortness of breath and coughing during exercise in healthy adults and more serious effects in the young, old, and infirm. Almost all of the research on ozone's effects has been done on lungs. There has not been any direct research on ozone and the sinuses. At the Air Pollution Health Effects Laboratory at the University of California, Irvine, however, its effects on the nasal cavities of rats have been studied. The findings lend substantial support to the connection between ozone and sinus disease. The researchers found significant damage to the mucous membrane surrounding the opening to the maxillary sinuses as a result of inhaling ozone. This could easily lead to the obstruction of the sinuses and subsequent infection. Robert Phalen, Ph.D., director of the laboratory, has also affirmed that "exposure to particulate pollution over a lifetime can be associated with increased infection and more exposure to diseases."

(Although not a part of the respiratory tract, the exposed surface of our eyes is covered by another mucous membrane called the conjunctiva. Eye irritation, burning, and tearing resulting from air pollution afflicts millions of people. Widely observed by eye doctors in the Los Angeles area, these symptoms are directly attributed to ozone. Although probably not quite as severe, particulates and the other pollutants can also cause similar symptoms. Dry air in combination with pollution can aggravate this condition even more.)

Nowhere in the United States is the problem of air pollution more acute than in Los Angeles. A recent study on a group of that city's ten- and eleven-year-olds revealed that their lung capacity is already diminished by 17 percent compared to the normal range for that age. A pathologist at the University of Southern California, in performing autopsies on Los Angeles children killed accidentally, has found a disturbing frequency of emphysematous changes previously seen only in adult lungs. But Los Angeles is not unique. Other areas of the country are well on their way to matching that city's severity of pollution and its damaging effects on the lungs and sinuses. There are also many agricultural communities that claim to be sinus "capitals" as a result of the pesticides and fertilizers that fill the air. I've heard from people in South Dakota, southern Minnesota, Iowa, North Carolina, and California's San Joaquin Valley, all reporting that "everyone has sinus problems." The residents of Dayton, Ohio, refer to their city as "Sinus Valley."

Most physicians would probably rate air pollution as the primary cause of the dramatic increase in the incidence of asthma, emphysema, chronic bronchitis (all have increased by 50 percent since 1981), and lung cancer. Americans are certainly not alone in suffering with this plague of pollution. According to the World Health Organization, residents of New Delhi, India; Seoul, Korea; and Mexico City breathe far worse air than that in Los Angeles. The air quality in many cities in eastern Europe is atrocious. Dying forests across central Europe are a testament to the air pollution of that heavily industrialized continent. Huge demonstrations demanding a cleanup of air pollution have been reported in many cities throughout the countries that formerly made up the Soviet Union.

There are solutions, of course, but most entail a change in lifestyle. In 1950, there were 50 million cars worldwide, 75 percent of them in the United States. This number doubled by 1960, redoubled by 1970, and doubled again by 1990—an eightfold increase to 400 million cars. American drivers now own only one-third of the world's total, but half of us have two cars in our garages. We have created a monster and it is killing us and the planet we live on. Automobiles, trucks, and buses are the chief sources of our air pollution. The availability and use of alternative fuels—ethanol, methanol, hydrogen, solar, and natural gas—or the electric car would make a profound difference. These fuels are domestic, cheaper, and more plentiful than gasoline. Greater enforcement of engine emission tests, development of mass transit systems, participation in carpooling, and construction of bicycle paths, along with the conversion of power plants from coal to natural gas, the development of solar energy, and a reduction in wood burning—all would have an immediate impact on cleaning our air.

Many of us are already suffering the ill effects of breathing unhealthy air. If the EPA is correct in concluding that air pollution is responsible for approximately 60,000 deaths a year, that would make it one of the leading causes of death in the United States. In a landmark eleven-year study completed in 1991 by the UCLA School of Medicine, it was proven that irreversible lung deterioration can result from chronic exposure to polluted air. According to the American Lung Association, annual medical costs associated with human exposure to all outdoor air pollutants from all sources range from $40 billion to $50 billion. If each of us will do at least one thing to decrease air pollution, collectively we can cure this plague of unhealthy air.

AIR POLLUTION: INDOOR

Unfortunately, we cannot escape dirty air by remaining indoors. In 1988 the EPA reported that indoor air can be as much as 100 times more polluted than outdoor air, noting that Americans spend 90 percent of their time indoors. All of the indoor air pollutants listed in Table 2-1 have been proved harmful to the respiratory tract. Some of these pollutants originate in outdoor air.

Sick building syndrome is an unscientific term used to describe a pattern of disease symptoms linked to poor indoor air quality in workplaces, schools, homes, and other buildings. A sick building is one in which at least 20 percent of the occupants experience discomfort that is suspected to be caused by contaminated indoor air. It need not be proven. The World Health Organization estimates that 30 percent of new or remodeled commercial buildings generate unusually high health and comfort complaints, and could be considered "sick buildings." Nationwide, as many as 80 million buildings might be of this type. Nearly a fifth of the work force in the United States has reported indoor air pollution ailments, ranging from headaches and fatigue to colds, influenza, and chronic respiratory illnesses (e.g., chronic sinusitis and chronic bronchitis). One million hospital visits a year are attributed to poor indoor air quality. According to John Sturdivant, president of the 700,000-member American Federation of Government Employees, "threats to health as a result of poor indoor air quality in the workplace have long been speculated. But as more and more of us experience sinus or nasal congestion, shortness of breath, and other symptoms, a pattern seems to be developing."

The EPA's own building in Washington, D.C., ironically, serves as an excellent example of sick building syndrome. Following renovations made to the building between 1987 and 1989, more than a thousand of the 5,500 employees at EPA headquarters have complained of headaches, rashes, nausea, fatigue, blurred vision, chills, sneezing, fever, irritability, forgetfulness, hoarseness, dizziness, and burning sensations in their throats, ears, eyes, and chests. One employee commented, "I was afraid I was going to die in the place." Several of these symptoms can be attributed to sick sinuses and chronically inflamed respiratory tracts.

Table 2-1

Indoor Air Pollutants

Automotive Fumes
Sources include outdoor traffic, outdoor parking lots, and outdoor loading and unloading spaces, as well as indoor garages

Chemicals and Chemical Solutions (chemicals that affect indoor air quality are those associated with architecture, the interior, artifacts, and maintenance)

Fungicides and pesticides in carpet-cleaning residues and sprays; formaldehyde used in the manufacture of insulation, plywood, fiberboard, furniture, and wood paneling; toxic solvents in oil-based paints, finishes, and wall sealants; aerosol sprays; office equipment chemicals, especially photocopiers and computers.

Combustion Products
Tobacco smoke★

Coal- or wood-burning fireplaces and stoves

Fuel combustion gases from gas-fired appliances such as ranges, clothes dryers, water heaters, and fireplaces (they produce nitrogen dioxide, carbon monoxide, nitrous oxides, sulfur oxides, hydrocarbons, and formaldehyde)

Ion Depletion or Imbalance
Too few negative ions

Excess of positive ions over negative ions

Microorganisms (primarily from humidifiers, air conditioners, and any other building components affected by excessive moisture)
Bacteria

Viruses

Molds

Dust mites (usually found in more humid areas)

Particulates
Dust

Pollen

Animal dander

Particles (frayed materials)

Asbestos

Radionuclides
Radon, a radioactive gas emitted from the earth that enters homes primarily through basements, crawl spaces, and water supply, especially from wells (it can attach to the particulates of cigarette smoke, dust particles, and natural aerosols)

A major explanation for the sick building syndrome, experts say, is the nationwide campaign, which emerged during the en-

---

★ From all of the available scientific data, tobacco smoke is the most unhealthy indoor air pollutant.

ergy crisis of the mid-1970s, to conserve energy by sealing and insulating buildings. The tight, energy efficient homes and buildings that evolved have a relatively low energy demand, but a correspondingly low ventilation rate. The demise of the operable-window building and the replacement of natural ventilation with mechanical ventilation have diminished the flow of fresh air, trapping pollutants inside. Furthermore, the fresh air in most cities is anything but fresh. There has also been an increase in the use of energy efficient heating and air-conditioning systems, which has often led to increased circulation of polluted indoor air. Another factor in the deterioration of indoor air quality is the type of materials used to construct and furnish buildings. Building materials and furniture made of petrochemical-based products and materials that can emit harmful chemical vapors over long periods of time are used in place of nonpolluting natural materials and fibers.

A fascinating aspect of this problem was revealed when several sick buildings were tested for the amount and type of ions present in the air. Areas having a high rate of employee complaints were found to have one of two ion conditions: (1) an abnormally low level of negative ions, or (2) an excess of positive ions compared to negative ions. When a more natural level of negative ions was reestablished through the use of negative-ion generators, the high complaint rate decreased dramatically. In energy efficient buildings, the constant recirculating of room air leads to a depletion of beneficial negative ions and often an increase in detrimental positive ions. The EPA spent hundreds of thousands of dollars trying to solve the problem of its sick headquarters, but the symptoms continued. On December 23, 1993, in Superior Court in the District of Columbia, five EPA employees were awarded $950,000 for ailments they said were related to unhealthy indoor air. There is a great deal that can be done to improve indoor air quality. Chapter 7 will offer many suggestions.

DRY AIR

An important function of the sinuses is to humidify the air we breathe; a person with weak sinuses may therefore have a problem in especially dry air. Moist air, that between 40 and 60 percent humidity, is very helpful for the proper functioning of the mucous membrane, especially the cilia. Dry air is usually found in conjunction with

- arid or semiarid climate;
- forced-air heating systems (they not only dry, but give the sinuses more to filter);
- air conditioning, especially in cars;
- oxygen therapy for various respiratory conditions;
- wind;
- mountains (the higher the elevation, the drier the air); and
- wood-burning stoves.

Dry air is hard on sinuses, but excessively moist air can also cause problems. Many microorganisms, such as bacteria, viruses, and molds, thrive when the humidity exceeds 60 percent.

COLD AIR

Although the moisture content of cold air is generally much higher than that of dry air, the shock of cold temperatures to the mucous membrane of an impaired nose and sinus can cause significant irritation and ciliary injury, and often results in at least a runny nose. Many of us are familiar with the constant mucus drip associated with cold weather activities such as ice skating, skiing, and snowmobiling. If you have chronic sinusitis or another respiratory condition, it is wise to take some precautions to protect your mucous membranes from cold air. In recent years it has been reported that many members of the Swedish cross-country ski team have developed adult-onset asthma due to their strenuous exercise in cold, dry air. The least stressful air temperatures on the respiratory tract are between 65° and 85°F.

ALLERGIES

Those with asthma and nasal allergies, also called hay fever, are very susceptible to sinus infections. Their nasal and sinus mucosae are extremely sensitive and often hyperactive and potentially hypersecretory. When an allergic reaction takes place there is swelling of the mucosa and obstruction of the sinuses. Although the theory is untested, I strongly believe that chronic breathing of polluted air heightens the sensitivity of the nasal mucosa, hence creating an increasing number of new allergy sufferers and worsening the allergic condition of many others. As yet, I haven't heard any other scientific explanation for the dramatic increase over the past decade in the number of people with allergies.

Many people claim that they are "allergic" to cigarette smoke, or dust, or some other irritant in the air. Most of the time they are not really describing an allergy, but rather an extreme irritation of the mucous membrane. This sensitivity causes a similar end result, nasal stuffiness and mucus drainage (and often a headache), but the process is a bit different. Actual nasal allergies are usually caused by airborne pollen from grass, trees, weeds, and flowers; molds; and dander from cats, dogs, horses, or other animals. In many areas of the United States, especially in parts of California and Florida where there is something pollinating year-round, allergies are the major contributors to sinus problems. Be aware, however, that if you are complaining of a year-round allergy problem, you might have chronic sinusitis.

In recent years an increasing number of physicians are recognizing that food allergies might be a factor in chronic sinusitis. The foods most often implicated are wheat, cow's milk and all other dairy products, chocolate, oranges, eggs, and artificial food coloring.

OCCUPATIONAL HAZARDS

A job performed in dirty, dry, and extremely hot or cold air should be considered a high risk to the sinuses. In recent years I have added high levels of positive ions as an additional risk factor. This applies especially to pilots and flight attendants, because of the high level of positive ions in aircraft cabin air, and to people who work in front of computer screens all day. In my experience, those at highest risk include

- auto mechanics,
- construction workers (especially carpenters, who are America's highest-risk group for ethmoid sinus cancer),
- painters,
- beauticians,
- airport and airline personnel (mechanics, maintenance workers, baggage handlers, flight attendants, and even pilots),
- white-collar workers in offices where there are one or more smokers, and who spend most of their time working with computers,
- policemen,
- firemen,
- parking garage attendants, and
- professional cyclists (the highest-risk group; they have more air to filter and are exposed to extremely cold, dry, and often dirty air).

When I worked as the team physician for the 7-Eleven cycling team during the 1986 Coors International Bicycle Classic, a total of five riders in the competition, including Eric Heiden of 7-Eleven, had to drop out because of sinus infections—this in spite of the fact that professional cyclists are the most physically fit human beings I have ever known.

DENTAL PROBLEMS

The roots of the upper teeth and the maxillary sinus are in close proximity; they are separated only by paper-thin bone or sinus mucosa. Because of this proximity, dental infections of the upper teeth can extend into the sinus cavity and cause maxillary sinusitis. It is also why toothache is a common symptom associated with maxillary sinusitis. Minor trauma or injury, dental instrumentation, extraction, or displacement of a chronically inflamed tooth can lead to perforation of the sinus cavity. The incidence of dental-related sinusitis in children is unknown but probably significant, particularly in adolescents. In adults, possibly 10 percent of maxillary sinus infections are thought to be of dental origin.

IMMUNODEFICIENCY

The immune system is the human body's natural defense against infection, cancer, or inflammation; indeed, any form of illness. Sometimes, for reasons medical science has been unable to explain, the immune system does not function normally. Vital components of this system are infection-fighting proteins called immunoglobulins. In immunodeficiency there is a decrease in the amount of one or two of these proteins. This condition can be diagnosed by a blood test. People who have a hereditary predisposition to it, who are on a course of chemotherapy, or who are taking cortisone long-term for a chronic condition are likely to have impaired immune systems. Most often, however, there is no known cause.

Other than air pollution, what may eventually prove to be the most significant cause of the epidemic of chronic sinusitis is the depressed immunity resulting from the overuse (long-term or repeated courses) of broad-spectrum antibiotics. This problem will be discussed in depth in Chapter 5.

MALFORMATIONS

Malformations include any physical problem that would result in the obstruction of the tiny sinus openings, the ostia. The most common malformations are a deviated septum (the wall that divides the two sides of the nose), enlarged adenoids (especially in young children), and polyps, cysts, or turbinate hypertrophy (swelling of the mucosal lining covering the internal nasal ridges).

A deviated septum is most often diagnosed by ear, nose, and throat surgeons as the primary cause of repeated sinus infections. In most instances, however, I strongly believe that this is not the case. The obstruction of the ostia by the deviated septum is usually a result of the *swollen mucosa* covering the septum and the turbinates of the opposite side of the nostril. If the cause of this swelling and inflammation is treated, then the surgery so often recommended by these surgeons becomes unnecessary. Remember, too, that most deviated septums have been present since birth. Sinus problems usually have not.

EMOTIONAL STRESS

Emotional stress is probably the single most important determinant in whether someone develops a sinus infection. All of the other factors described in this chapter have the potential to adversely affect the sinuses, but what is it that triggers that potential? Why is it that a person with weak sinuses can be exposed to the same "risky" conditions many times but only occasionally develop a sinus infection? I am convinced that the answer is usually stress.

In the past few years, the new science of psychoneuroimmunology has legitimized the old notion that thoughts and emotions can both cause and combat disease. Recent research has provided a wealth of information on the profound impact our thoughts, beliefs, feelings, and attitudes have on our immune system and on our health. This knowledge is not new to holistic medicine. You will find its application to the treatment of sinus disease in Part II.

Chapter 3

RECOGNIZING A SICK SINUS: ACUTE AND CHRONIC

T hroughout this book I use the term *sinusitis* to refer to sinus problems in general. This word actually means "inflammation of a sinus" and encompasses two distinctly different medical diagnoses: acute sinusitis and chronic sinusitis. The criteria for these diagnoses, as they are presented in this chapter, have been jointly established by myself and Bruce Jafek, M.D., chairman of the Department of Otolaryngology at the University of Colorado School of Medicine.

ACUTE SINUSITIS

Acute sinusitis is another way of saying **sinus infection.** This is the problem that usually requires medical attention. I have already mentioned that the common cold is most often the cause of a sinus infection, so let's look at this a bit more closely.

The Common Cold
A person who has had negligible or no sinus problems previously will notice that after seven to ten days a cold still won't quit, or that the cold symptoms have actually gotten much worse, or that the cold was almost gone for one or two weeks and now it's back

again. Close questioning reveals that the "cold" never really went away.

Each of these scenarios is becoming much more commonplace. As I have previously mentioned, one recent study has revealed that 87 percent of those people who thought they just had a cold actually had an infected sinus as revealed by a CT scan —the most diagnostic test for sinusitis.

Just what is a cold? It is a viral infection of the nasal and usually sinus mucous membranes that is often immediately preceded by a sore throat. The primary symptoms are a stuffy and runny nose with thin clear or white mucus, fatigue, and mild muscle aching. Secondary symptoms might include headache, persistent sore throat, cough, and a low-grade fever. The average cold lasts from four to seven days.

In people whose sinuses have been weakened by previous infections, the common cold causes problems more quickly. These patients might notice the symptoms of a sinus infection within two or three days of the onset of the cold. The underlying condition of the sinuses will usually determine how soon the symptoms appear. Keep in mind that a common cold very often precedes the onset of acute sinusitis. Its appearance in the history of one's illness will help in the diagnosis of acute sinusitis. The most common symptoms follow. Note that the symptoms might differ for children under age twelve.

Head Congestion

Most people describe this symptom as fullness or a stuffy head. The nose might be stuffy as well. This symptom is most obvious in the morning upon arising from bed. It is often relieved, although not eliminated, by a hot shower. Voice, smell, and taste might be altered. These symptoms, however, are more subtle than the primary one of head congestion. There is a very definite awareness of a fullness in the head or a dull ache behind or above the eyes. *Dizziness* and *lightheadedness* are other words that might be used to describe this symptom.

Headache and Facial Pain

I have combined these two symptoms because it is often difficult to differentiate between them. With acute sinusitis, pain, and sometimes swelling, will occur in the region of the affected sinus (Figure 3-1). This usually results from air, pus, and mucus being trapped within the obstructed sinus. An infected maxillary sinus will cause pain, and sometimes swelling, in the cheek. Pain might occur under the eye and in the upper teeth, particularly the molars. At times, the *toothache* can be so severe as to prompt a visit to the dentist. When air is prevented from entering a sinus by a swollen mucous membrane at its opening, a vacuum can be created, also resulting in severe pain in the affected sinus. This is why many sinus sufferers experience pain with the barometric pressure changes related to weather systems (low pressure), and while descending (prior to landing) in an airplane.

Infected ethmoid sinuses produce pain between and behind the eyes, and tenderness when pressure is applied to the sides of the nose. Infected frontals cause pain in the forehead and over the eyes. Infected sphenoids produce a generalized pain, deep in the head, which becomes aggravated whenever your head is jarred. Sphenoid pain is often perceived as a headache in the back of the head at the base of the skull.

Children might experience facial pain accompanied by swelling of the orbit of the eye that involves the upper eyelid. Gradual in onset, the swelling is most obvious in the early morning, shortly after rising. The swelling might decrease or even disappear during the day, only to reappear the following day. Children might also experience photophobia, which is an unwillingness to open the eyes in bright light.

Some of the most incapacitating headaches I have seen resulted from infected frontal sinuses. Sinus headaches tend to worsen when you bend your head forward or lie down, and tend to be worse in the morning, after you have been in bed for hours, and then ease somewhat later in the day.

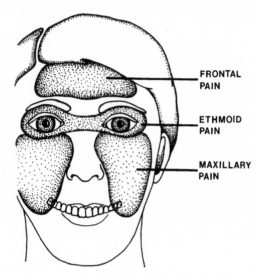

FIGURE 3-1.   *Location of Sinus Pain in Acute Sinusitis*

Extreme Fatigue

There is scarcely a sinus patient I can think of who doesn't complain of some degree of fatigue. Most people, even if they are not ill, would admit to being tired for some part of the day. The word *extreme* in regard to fatigue means a definite change in normal energy level.

In addition to inquiring about the nasal and head symptoms that are usually mentioned by the patient, I always ask the questions, "Does your whole body feel sick in some way?" and "Do you feel especially tired?" The answer to these questions is frequently yes because acute sinusitis is usually a systemic illness, one that affects the entire body. These patients are sick all over. The medical term that best describes this phenomenon is *malaise,* meaning a feeling of general discomfort. It is often accompanied by significant irritability. People with sinus infections are usually sleeping more at night than they normally would, having some difficulty getting through a full day at work, and perhaps even taking unaccustomed naps. In people who exercise regularly, the drop in energy level is even more evident.

At times, fatigue is the chief complaint. The bad cold someone had was as long ago as two or three months, and they say, "I just haven't been myself since." These people do not come in complaining of the cold they still have; most of the time they think they are finished with it. If asked, however, they will admit to a stuffy head in the morning and occasional yellow mucus they have to spit out. These patients pose a tough diagnostic challenge to the physician, as some of them have been tired for so long they have no recollection of any previous illness. Others have been misdiagnosed with anything from depression to menopause. A few days of antibiotics, however, can do what months of estrogen or an antidepressant were unable to do.

Yellow Mucus

The question that seems to make patients most uncomfortable is "What color is your mucus?" The usual response, accompanied by a grimace, is "Eww, I never look at it!" The classic presentation of acute sinusitis in children, less frequently seen in an adult, is yellow (actually a yellow-green) mucus coming from one nostril. If it's not (no pun intended), the diagnosis may be difficult. Most kids are not great nose-blowers, but sniffing actually makes matters worse, in that it tends to suck bacteria into the sinus. I usually try to have young patients blow their noses in the examination room. If you are checking your child at home, please remember to use white tissues; yellow won't help at all. Sinusitis is often missed in children. An article several years ago in a pediatric journal stated that almost 25 percent of all diagnosed upper respiratory tract infections (the common cold) in kids were actually cases of acute sinusitis. In light of the recent study revealing 87 percent of adults with "colds" were, in fact, suffering from sinus infections, I would speculate that there is a similar high percentage in children as well.

In adults, yellow mucus from the nose will help make the diagnosis. However, in many cases the mucus is either clear or white, or there is none at all from the nose. It seems that in most adult cases of acute sinusitis the infected or yellow mucus drains down the back of the throat. People are most aware of this in the morning, when they get out of bed and spit into the sink some of the mucus their sinuses have produced during the night. This morning yellow mucus is helpful in making the diagnosis but it can also be present in the absence of acute sinusitis. Therefore, the most important question I ask an adult is, "Are you spitting out yellow mucus during the rest of the day, other than first thing in the morning?" (It is the consistent, all-day colored mucus that is most definitive in making the diagnosis.) Unfortunately, most people will respond with "I swallow it," or "It's not convenient to spit it out," or the old standby, "I never look at it!" If I still suspect a sinus infection, I will ask if they are even aware of mucus dripping down the back of the throat. If they're not aware of this occurring during the day, I then ask, "How about when you wake up in the morning?" Often I see patients who aren't aware of mucus drainage, but when I look at their throats, there is a thick yellow band of mucus running down from their sinuses.

I've spent a lot of time on the topic of mucus not because I enjoy discussing "gross" subjects, as my daughter Julie would say, but because it is extremely helpful in making the diagnosis. There are very few objective, or visible, signs of acute sinusitis, but this one is consistently present.

Refining the Diagnosis

Most ear, nose, and throat (ENT) specialists would find yellow mucus too indefinite a finding with which to make a diagnosis. Until 1986, they usually attempted to confirm the diagnosis with a sinus X-ray. However, this is unreliable. Some patients will have every symptom of a sinus infection although an X-ray shows a normal sinus.

Since then, new technology has made the definitive diagnosis of acute sinusitis much more feasible. The CT ("cat") scan, a computerized tomographic X-ray technique, can show areas of the sinuses never clearly visible with conventional X-rays. As a

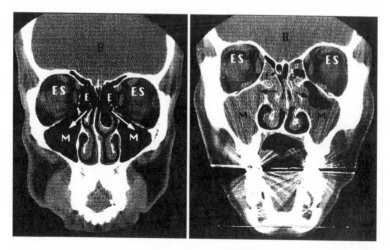

Figure 3-2. *CT ("CAT") SCAN   Severely diseased sinuses (markedly thickened lining) are seen on the right with normal sinus computed tomogram (CT) x-ray on the left for comparison. The maxillary (cheek)(labeled M) and ethmoid (between eye sockets)(E) sinuses are seen here with the brain (B) and eye sockets (ES) for anatomical reference. The arrows on the right clearly show the blockage of the outflow (osteomeatal complex) of the ethmoid and maxillary sinuses on the right with a clear opening on the patient on the left.*

result, the diagnosis of sinus disease, and correspondingly, the statistics on its incidence, have risen dramatically. Unfortunately, the average sinus CT scan is costly, and not very convenient.

To help reduce medical costs—as well as to assist primary care physicians, allergists, and ENT specialists in treating sinus infections—it would be a great advantage to have a generally accepted clinical diagnosis of acute sinusitis. Together with Dr. Jafek, this is what we are offering here: a list of signs and symptoms that are so often present with sinus infections that they will preclude the need for X-rays and other expensive diagnostic procedures.

The picture presented by acute sinusitis can vary greatly; some people are very sick, others minimally uncomfortable. However, you can usually depend on these elements to make a definitive clinical diagnosis in an adult: *a preceding cold, head congestion, head-*

ache, extreme fatigue, and postnasal yellow mucus. In a child the most common symptoms are nasal yellow mucus, fever, foul-smelling breath, and cough.

More Diagnostic Clues
The following symptoms are not quite as consistent as the foregoing, but are frequently present.

Fever A high temperature accompanying sinusitis is much more common in children than in adults. When fever is present in an adult, it is usually less than 101°F. It is not uncommon to see kids run high fevers (as high as 103° to 105°F) with acute sinusitis. Fever often appears early in the course of the infection—when other symptoms are not yet obvious—making the diagnosis difficult. Because fever accompanies so many different infections, it can't be considered an important diagnostic symptom. However, if I suspect sinusitis, fever, along with the other symptoms, can be a helpful sign in confirming the diagnosis.

Nasal Congestion and Rhinorrhea A stuffy and runny nose (rhinorrhea) is a primary symptom of the common cold that usually precedes acute sinusitis. The two infections very often overlap. The important thing to remember in adult sinusitis is that stuffiness is more common than a runny nose and is often present on only one side of the nose. In children with sinusitis, the yellow nasal discharge can be copious. With a cold, draining mucus is usually clear or white and thin or watery. With sinusitis it is usually thick and yellow.

Sore Throat A sore throat is probably the most common complaint in any family doctor's office. The underlying problem is not always sinusitis, but a substantial number of sore throats do result from mouth breathing and from postnasal mucus drainage down the back of the throat. A sore throat from sinusitis is usually not consistent throughout the day; it is much worse in the morning upon awakening. In fact, the soreness, caused by constant postnasal mucus drainage, a stuffy nose, and mouth breathing can keep people from sleeping through the night. The dry air most of us breathe in our bedrooms can be irritating, too. Once I have established that a patient's sore throat is much worse first thing in the morning, I ask if the patient is aware of mucus draining down the back of the throat. (In children, this drainage often results in bad breath.) After that, I merely have to run through a checklist of the other sinus symptoms—mucus color, recent cold, fatigue, fever, and so on—to decide if this is sinusitis or something else. Most of these questions would be asked as part of a thorough investigation of any sore throat.

Laryngitis Laryngitis, or hoarseness, is another common symptom of sinus infection. It results from the same factors that cause sore throat, primarily postnasal mucus draining down into the larynx, causing irritation, inflammation, and swelling of the vocal cords and the arytenoid cartilages in the larynx.

Cough For most of the patients who come to a family doctor's office with a sinus infection, cough and sore throat are the symptoms that have resulted in the greatest discomfort and the most loss of sleep. Unfortunately, they are also the symptoms that have resulted in the highest number of misdiagnoses. A cough might be mistaken for bronchitis. Why? Because the cough of a sinusitis patient comes from yellow mucus draining down the back of the throat and continuing into the trachea or upper airway. Most physicians are aware that a productive cough that brings up a purulent or yellow mucus is often bronchitis. It isn't unusual to make that diagnosis in spite of hearing clear lungs with the stethoscope. It is easy to understand this common mistake, but it is just as easy to ask a few simple questions to rule out bronchitis and rule in acute sinusitis.

The cough from a sinus infection in adults isn't usually too bad during the day, when they are upright, but often worsens as soon as they lie down in bed at night. In children, the cough tends to be persistent throughout the day, just as it is in adults with bronchitis. Adults usually swallow the postnasal mucus drainage unconsciously, while up and about. This gets the mucus away from the trachea and into the stomach. (Swallowing the mucus can result in another not uncommon symptom that accompanies sinus infections: gastrointestinal upset; i.e., abdominal discomfort and loose bowels. There might be two or three loose movements a day—not quite diarrhea, but a definite change in bowel pattern. However, this isn't nearly as common as other symptoms I've mentioned, so I apologize for getting off the tract—respiratory, that is. Now, back to the cough.)

After asking about the timing of the cough, I usually want to know, "Does the cough feel like it's deep in your chest or does it feel more like a tickle in the back of your throat?" The latter, a dry cough, is much more typical of sinusitis; whereas the former, a wet, mucusy cough, is more indicative of bronchitis. In the past few years, I have noticed a definite increase in the number of patients who are infected simultaneously in the sinuses and lungs. This is called sinobronchitis. If the antibiotic treatments for sinusitis and bronchitis were the same, there would be no need to differentiate between the two. However, this is not the case, and I believe it is valuable to be as specific as possible in a treatment program.

I began this chapter by describing acute sinusitis as an infection usually requiring medical attention. A visit to the doctor has a twofold purpose: to diagnose the problem and to begin treating it. Ideally, there should also be a third objective: education and prevention. That is, teaching the patient how to care for his sinuses so that future office visits for the same problem will be unnecessary.

Again, the recognition of acute sinusitis is not a simple matter, even for physicians. Because the condition can manifest itself differently from one time to the next, this chapter and the next should be referred to frequently.

CHRONIC SINUSITIS

According to the 1992 National Health Interview Survey, administered jointly by the Centers for Disease Control and Prevention and the National Center for Health Statistics, *chronic sinusitis is the most common chronic disease in the United States.* For all ages, it afflicts nearly 15 percent, or one out of every seven people in this country. That's approximately 40 million people. When the same study was performed in 1989, just less than 14 percent of all Americans had the problem. For some reason, it is more common in women than men, reaching its peak incidence among middle-aged women. Twenty-two percent of all women between the ages of forty-five and sixty-four have chronic sinusitis (15 percent of men in this age group have it), about equal with the incidence of high blood pressure (hypertension). This makes it second only to arthritis among the most common chronic diseases for women this age. In men of this age group, it ranks fourth, behind high blood pressure, hearing impairment, and arthritis.

Although sinus disease has reached epidemic proportions, most people who have chronic sinusitis couldn't tell you they do. Their situation is similar to that of the hundreds of thousands of people who are unaware they have hypertension or diabetes, two other common chronic conditions. They may be experiencing some of the symptoms of these ailments but are unable to attach a label or diagnosis to their problem. However, what the vast majority of these sinus sufferers are very familiar with are tissues and handkerchiefs, postnasal drip, congestion, headaches, fatigue, irritability, halitosis, a weak sense of smell and taste, and to an increasing extent, frequent courses of antibiotics and even sinus surgery.

Chronic sinusitis can be either:

1. a persistent low-grade infection with periodic flare-ups of acute sinusitis These people are always sick to some degree. It may have been many months, and in most cases years, since they've been healthy, or completely normal. Their chronic illness takes the form of an ongoing sinus infection with any or all of the symptoms I've previously described for acute sinusitis. Extreme fatigue, headaches, and persistent yellow-green post-nasal mucus drainage top the list of a multitude of systemic (total body) symptoms usually present in these sinus sufferers. They have taken multiple ten-day or two-week courses of powerful broad-spectrum antibiotics, and have often undergone multiple sinus surgeries, with minimal to moderate improvement in their symptoms. But the sinus infection never totally clears up. (One sure sign of a lingering infection is persistent yellow-green mucus drainage.) Some of these people in group 1 have been on continuous antibiotics for months, and in some cases a year or more. I know of one woman who has had fourteen sinus surgeries. These people constitute the majority of the patients I've treated during the past three years. They are often frustrated, angry, depressed, and they feel chronically ill. Their physicians share their exasperation. Conventional medicine has done all it can do for them, and to no avail.

2. recurrent or repeated sinus infections (acute sinusitis) These people suffer at least three or more infections within a six-month period. They usually have most of the symptoms I've already described for each episode of acute sinusitis. However, they often do not have a cold before their sinus infection begins. What might have started out as a cold in someone with healthier mucous membranes becomes an almost immediate sinus infection with an accompanying prescription for an antibiotic, in most of the members of group 2. Following the course of antibiotic treatment and between infections, these people usually feel okay or almost "normal." Their normal condition, however, may now include frequent sinus headaches, a stuffy nose and head, a somewhat diminished energy level, chronic postnasal drip (white or clear mucus), and increased irritability.

3. chronic inflammation with little or no infection These people are not nearly as sick or uncomfortable as those in groups 1 and 2. They have chronic inflammation of the mucous membranes lining their nose and sinuses with infrequent (one or two per year) or no infections at all. Inflammation involves pain, swelling, and increased secretions from the mucous membrane, but without the causative agents of bacteria, viruses, or fungi that are present with infection. Most of the people in group 3 do not realize they have a treatable disease called chronic sinusitis, and usually do not seek medical attention. For those who have, many have heard from their doctors, "There's nothing that can be done for you." A more accurate statement would have been "There's nothing that I can do for you."

As a result, the majority have learned to accept their condition and have adjusted to a compromised quality of life that includes: head and nasal congestion, headaches, a runny nose and/or postnasal drip, increased irritability, halitosis, and possibly a diminished sense of smell and taste. Chronic sinus sufferers usually have an increased sensitivity to the factors mentioned in Chapter 2, such as cigarette smoke, pollution, dryness, cold, and fumes. The more they are exposed to any one of these irritants, the more pronounced the symptoms will be, and the more often they are likely to develop acute sinus infections. Although most of these symptoms are similar for all three groups of chronic sinusitis, they are usually less severe in group 3. The majority of the members of the first two groups of chronic sinus sufferers began in group 3. After a gradual weakening of their mucous membrane due to chronic inflammation, and a corresponding decrease in their natural resistance to infection (a normal mucosa protects against infection), colds become more frequent. These are often followed by sinus infections, and the cycle escalates to weaker membranes and more infections, more antibiotics, and a subsequently weaker immune system. The common cold becomes a rare occurrence and almost every illness, whether it begins as influenza, strep throat, or stomach flu, eventually seems to end up as a sinus infection. Unless the cycle can be broken, the immune system remains depressed and the sinuses are left in a permanently weak and damaged state.

Almost everyone who has made at least a two-month commitment to practicing the Sinus Survival Program, described in Part II, considers themselves to be either cured of chronic sinusitis or to have returned to group 3. For many of these "sinus survivors," their ongoing or chronic symptoms may be so negligible that it is difficult to make a distinction between being cured and being a type 3. They may not be aware of any symptoms at all unless they have developed a sinus infection. Just as with groups 1 and 2, there is a spectrum of severity of symptoms and degrees of discomfort. Usually, the longer a person adheres to the Sinus Survival Program, the more mild a type 3 they become. If there are no persistent symptoms but the individual still has one or two episodes of acute sinusitis during the year, I would consider that person to be cured of chronic sinusitis.

There are other methods of classification. Some physicians label anyone who has had an infection of the sinuses lasting three months or more as suffering from chronic sinusitis. But I believe that this is too limited a definition to account for the 40 million chronic sinus sufferers identified by the National Health Interview Survey.

The nose and sinuses have become the "weak spot" in the bodies of people with chronic sinusitis. Although not a life-threatening illness, chronic sinusitis affects its victims daily as an energy-draining condition that can have a profound impact on their ability to enjoy life. However, as the gateway and defender of the lungs, the nose and sinuses have a vital function to perform. As millions of sick sinuses fail to protect the lungs by filtering out bacteria, viruses, pollutants, and pollen, and are unable to humidify and warm dry and cold air adequately, we are beginning to experience an epidemic of life-threatening lung disease.

TABLE 3-1

Diagnosing and Recognizing the Symptoms of Colds, Sinusitis, and Allergies

Primary Symptoms—almost always present
Secondary Symptoms—frequent but less often present

THE COMMON COLD

Primary:
- preceded by high stress; too much going on at once
- preceded by a sore throat
- nasal congestion
- runny nose
- thin clear/white nasal mucus
- fatigue
- mild muscle aching
- lasts for four to seven days

Secondary:
- headache
- sore throat
- cough
- low-grade fever

SINUS INFECTION (ACUTE SINUSITIS)

Primary:
- preceded by the common cold
- preceded by unexpressed anger
- head congestion (facial or head fullness)
- head or facial pain (headache, cheek, tooth, or eye pain)
- thick green/yellow nasal or especially postnasal mucus drainage (down back of throat)
- extreme fatigue
- lasts for two or more weeks

Secondary:
- preceded by allergies or by prolonged exposure to air pollution, smoke, or toxic fumes
- fever

- sore throat
- cough
- hoarseness
- nasal congestion
- lasts for several months

ALLERGIES, HAY FEVER, OR ALLERGIC RHINITIS

Primary:

- preceded by personal or family history of allergies, eczema, or asthma
- intermittent symptoms: either seasonal (pollen), food-related, environmentally or emotionally triggered
- positive allergy skin tests
- thin, clear/white nasal mucus
- nasal congestion
- sneezing
- itching of nose, eyes, or throat
- symptoms relieved with antihistamines, food elimination, environmental clearing, or stress reduction

Secondary:

- persistent or perennial symptoms
- postnasal drip with intermittent sore throat, cough, or hoarseness
- wheezing, difficulty breathing
- skin rash
- allergic "shiners" (dark circles under eyes)

Chapter 4

IDENTIFYING THE OTHER COMMON RESPIRATORY DISEASES: ALLERGIES, ASTHMA, AND BRONCHITIS

According to the most recent report from the National Center for Health Statistics, there are now four respiratory conditions among the ten most common chronic diseases in the United States. Besides chronic sinusitis in the number-one position (afflicting more than 38 million people or nearly 15 percent of our population), allergic rhinitis, or hay fever, is number five (affecting more than 10 percent), while chronic bronchitis (5.4 percent) and asthma (4.9 percent) are the eighth and ninth most common chronic conditions. In 1982 these percentages were 12.1 for sinusitis, 8.5 for allergies, 3.4 for bronchitis, and 3.5 for asthma. In 1970, of these four respiratory ailments, only hay fever was among the top ten. I have documented this information not only because I enjoy statistics, but also because in some instances statistics can be quite revealing. In this case, there is incontrovertible evidence that the health of our respiratory tracts is deteriorating and our subsequent ability to breathe is being threatened.

These four chronic respiratory conditions all affect a part of the same tract (refer to Figure 1-2, on page 5). The nose, sinuses, and lungs are anatomically connected by the airway, histologically (refers to "tissues") joined by one continuous respiratory epithelial lining, and intimately related by their sharing of mucus from one cavity to another. It should come as no surprise then that these common respiratory ailments often occur sequentially or in some cases almost simultaneously. For instance, if you suffer from hay fever and your nose is really stuffed up, this can easily close off the ostia (the opening of the sinus ducts), prevent the sinuses from draining, and create the ideal conditions for a sinus infection to occur. Once you have a sinus infection, it isn't difficult to imagine the bacteria in the infected mucus draining from the sinuses down the back of your throat and infecting your lungs, triggering either asthma, bronchitis, or both.

ASTHMA

There are, of course, statistics to support the phenomenon of the interrelatedness of sinusitis and asthma. The National Jewish Center for Immunology and Respiratory Medicine in Denver, a research center for asthma and other respiratory diseases, noted in a 1989 study that more than two-thirds of patients with mild to severe asthma showed abnormalities on sinus X-rays. It was also reported that in asthmatic children with moderate to severe sinus abnormalities, treatment of their sinuses may improve their asthma. The study postulated two mechanisms to explain how sinus disease could cause asthma: postnasal drip of mucus into the lower airways, which either directly alters airway reactivity or causes airway inflammation; and nasal obstruction, which causes mouth breathing, aggravating the asthma through loss of heat and moisture in the lower airways, particularly if the air breathed is cold and dry.

The National Jewish Center primarily treats asthmatics whose condition is poorly controlled or who depend on cortisone to control the asthma. The center's study linking sinus disease to asthma described many patients who improved dramatically and were able to decrease their steroid requirements following treatment of their sinusitis. This has been demonstrated by other studies and is now a well-accepted principle in the treatment of asthma. If this holds true for the most severely afflicted asthmatics, it should also apply to anyone with mild to moderate asthma who experiences a flare-up or an exacerbation of the condition. If an obvious cause of the asthmatic episode is not present—such as the common cold, allergy, exercise, or emotional stress—and the wheezing can't be controlled with the usual medication, consider the possibility of a sinus infection.

Asthma is the most frightening and life-threatening of the common respiratory conditions. *Its primary symptom is difficult breathing,* with or without an audible wheeze, cough, a constricted chest, or painfully congested lungs. Affecting the small airways, called bronchioles, asthma causes swelling of the respiratory mucosa lining the airway, thicker and increased mucus secretion into the airway, and contraction of the smooth muscle lining the bronchiolar walls. These three obstructive changes occurring together leave very little room for air to pass through. In addition to airway obstruction, asthma is also characterized by airway inflammation. This, in turn, causes airway hyperresponsiveness resulting in a heightened sensitivity to airborne allergens, pollutants, and cold and dry air.

Asthma is now considered an epidemic of its own, with the number of asthmatics in the United States more than doubling since 1980 to more than 13 million. In spite of the fact that available treatment is better than it has ever been, the death rate has also doubled since 1980; 5,000 Americans now die from asthma each year. Although its incidence is relatively equal among all age groups, more children than ever before are dying from asthma, and those at greatest risk are boys, blacks, and urban children. It is the number-one reason for children missing school. The estimated annual costs of asthma therapy in this country approach $11 billion. That includes the direct cost of physicians' time, hospitalization charges, and medications, and the indirect costs to patients, families, and their employers for lost work time.

Although asthma has been described by physicians for hundreds of years, no one within the medical community is willing to state conclusively the cause for the dramatic increase in both the prevalence and severity of this condition. Similar increases have been noted in other countries, including Canada, Great Britain, France, Denmark, and Germany. Some researchers suspect increased air pollution or a heightened sensitivity to some allergens. Separate studies in New York, Connecticut, New Jersey, and Georgia from 1988 to 1990 all confirmed a strong association between the ozone levels in smog and the severity of asthma. On days when ozone levels were highest, asthma attacks increased by 30 percent and asthma admissions to hospitals increased by 25 to 30 percent. Ozone is known to inflame air passages, and swollen airways are one of the chief symptoms of asthma. A Canadian study in 1991 suggests that ozone can increase the lungs' responsiveness to allergens, such as ragweed or grass. Based on that research, it was recommended that during periods of high ozone, asthmatics should be inactive, stay inside, and use air conditioners.

Asthma has always been difficult to diagnose in infants and preschool children because they have trouble following directions for breathing-function tests. These tests are easier to administer to older children and adults and they can provide the definitive medical diagnosis. However, most people with asthma relate a history of the onset of their symptoms that can also provide a dependable diagnosis. Shortness of breath, coughing, wheezing, chest congestion, constriction, or pain following the onset of a cold, sinus infection, hay fever symptoms, emotional stress, or exercise are all common descriptions of asthma. In fact, exercise can trigger wheezing and shortness of breath in up to 80 percent of individuals who have been diagnosed with asthma, and 70 percent require treatment for their symptoms. According to the *Guidelines for the Diagnosis and Management of Asthma,* published by the National Institutes of Health, exercise-induced asthma should be anticipated in all asthma patients. I would add that asthmatics who exercise outdoors in highly polluted cities (especially with ozone and particulates), in cold temperatures, or on days with high pollen counts are at even greater risk of inducing an asthma attack. Needless to say, if you are an asthmatic and you have a sinus infection, I would postpone your workout, whether it's outdoors or indoors.

Although asthma was once regarded as a psychological malady, it is now seen by the medical community as a hereditary, immune system disorder that is sometimes linked to allergies. However, just as with any chronic disease, there are multiple causes, and one of them is always emotional. Asthma is no exception. There is a strong emotional component contributing to its cause that will be explored in greater depth in Part II.

ALLERGIC RHINITIS

Human beings, along with most other mammals, are meant to breathe through their noses. When a stuffy nose prevents us from doing so, it can be very unpleasant and uncomfortable. Nasal congestion is the most frequent and possibly the most troublesome symptom of allergies or hay fever. It results from the swelling and inflammation of the nasal mucous membrane. This inflammation is the key factor in causing hyperreactivity of the nasal mucosa, resulting in the other common nasal allergy symptoms of sneezing and itching. The sneezing usually occurs in a rapid, multiple sequence, and the itching might include the eyes as well. A thin, clear mucus drainage is also usually present with allergies (refer to Table 3-1, on pages 43–44).

It has nothing to do with hay and rarely produces a fever, but hay fever still makes about 27 million Americans miserable on an annual basis. Most people with allergies are sensitive to pollen—either tree, grass, or ragweed—and they make up the largest group of allergy sufferers. (North America is host to seventeen species of ragweed.) Their symptoms are seasonal, with tree pollen usually most plentiful from March to May, grasses from May to July, and ragweed from August to October. These seasons vary according to your locale and weather conditions. If the highly allergic person also has asthma, then the same pollen or allergens that trigger the nasal symptoms can also precipitate an asthmatic attack.

In addition to pollen, there are many other substances that can cause allergic rhinitis on a perennial or year-round basis. Among the most difficult to avoid are dust mites, microscopic insects that thrive by the millions wherever dust collects in a house. They live on shed human skin cells and leave droppings that are about the size of pollen grains, and just as easy to inhale. The mites prefer the warm, humid climates of coastal cities—New Orleans is high on the list of offenders in the United States—but they are very rare in cities above 6,000 feet, where the air is dry.

Mold spores can be found on food, leather, furniture, and in air conditioners. Outdoors, they can grow on crops, grass, and dead leaves. There can be hundreds of thousands of mold spores per cubic meter of air, and we inhale about 10 to 12 cubic meters of air each day. Unfortunately, these spores cause significant allergic reactions in millions of people.

About 25 percent of allergy sufferers are allergic to cats. The offending substance is the cat's saliva, which is left on their fur during preening. Homes with cats can be so full of cat hair and dander that it can take up to six months after the cat is removed before it can be considered safe for someone who is allergic to cats.

There are a multitude of foods that can cause allergy symptoms. Surveys have shown that as many as 70 percent of Americans believe they are allergic to at least one particular food. Yet a food allergy may be one of the most under-diagnosed conditions in this country because scientific testing has been inaccurate, it is expensive, and it demands carefully informed patients and technicians. As I've already explained, allergic rhinitis with its persistent nasal congestion can cause sinus infections, and a significant percentage of the allergic symptoms are probably caused by food. If you suspect a food allergy, then I would suggest a food–elimination diet to confirm the diagnosis. Eliminate from your diet for at least three weeks the foods that are most likely to produce nasal allergy symptoms: cow's milk and all dairy products, wheat, rye, oats, chocolate, corn, oranges, eggs, and artificial food coloring. After that, begin to introduce each of these foods into your diet at the rate of one every three days. It should be obvious to you which foods cause your nose to react.

Allergy skin tests are medicine's most definitive method of

diagnosing the cause of allergic rhinitis from airborne substances such as pollen, animal dander, etc. They involve injecting bits of suspected allergens in different places under the skin, or applying them to scratches on the arm or the back. If a particular area swells, reddens, and itches, the patient more often than not is allergic to that substance.

Most physicians agree that allergies result from aberrant functioning of the immune system, and that they tend to run in families. But there is no mention within the medical community of an emotional component causing allergies, nor is there any explanation for the tremendous increase in the number of allergy sufferers in the past fifteen years. My "sandpaper" theory holds that as we breathe polluted and particulate-laden air 23,000 times a day, we are causing chronic irritation ("rubbing the surface raw") and inflammation of the nasal mucous membrane. This creates a hyperreactive membrane that, given the right genetic predisposition, emotional stress, and adequate exposure to an allergen, can precipitate a lifetime of allergies.

CHRONIC BRONCHITIS

Bronchitis can be either an infection (acute bronchitis) or an inflammation (chronic bronchitis) of the bronchi, the two large tubes that branch off into the lungs from the windpipe (trachea). (Refer to Figure 4-1, page 52.) I have often seen acute bronchitis occur in conjunction with acute sinusitis. This condition is called sinobronchitis—an infection of both sinuses and lungs caused by the postnasal drainage of infected mucus into the lungs. Other than the usual symptoms of a sinus infection, there is also a persistent (day and night), deep, wet, and yellow mucusy cough. Another common respiratory condition is the coexistence of bronchitis with asthma, called asthmatic bronchitis. People are generally very sick with this condition and experience great difficulty breathing, while wheezing, coughing, and battling an infection in their lungs.

Chronic bronchitis is a condition in which excessive mucus is

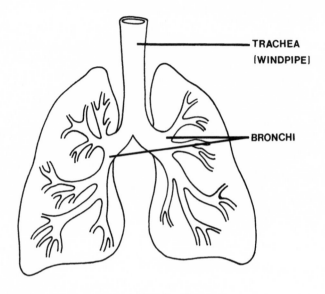

Figure 4-1. *Lungs*

secreted from the inflamed respiratory mucosa lining the bronchi. To qualify as chronic bronchitis, there must be a cough that produces thick white or gray mucus for at least three months, and the cough must recur for at least two consecutive years (according to the American Lung Association). In addition, there may be shortness of breath and wheezing, similar to the breathing problems experienced by people with asthma. This latter condition is referred to as chronic asthmatic bronchitis.

In addition to the cough and wheezing, other frequent symptoms of chronic bronchitis include difficulty breathing, frequent episodes of acute bronchitis, weakness, and weight loss.

The typical person with chronic bronchitis is forty-five years of age or older. It is significantly more common in women than men. The chief cause is cigarette smoking, but smoking marijuana in lesser amounts than cigarettes can produce similar lung damage. Repeated attacks of acute bronchitis may also lead to chronic bronchitis. People, especially smokers, who live in highly polluted cities are even more susceptible to the disease, as are those with other chronic lung diseases such as asthma and emphysema. Occupational exposure to dust or toxic fumes can also increase the risk of chronic bronchitis. A recent study published in the November 1994 *Journal of the American Medical Association* has shown that quitting smoking can repair some of the lung damage causing chronic bronchitis.

Specific diagnostic studies such as a sputum analysis and lung function tests are used to confirm the diagnosis of chronic bronchitis. Tests are also needed to exclude other diseases that may cause similar symptoms, such as silicosis, tumors in the upper airway, or even tuberculosis (TB). The chief symptoms of TB are a persistent cough, fatigue, and weight loss.

Tuberculosis was this country's primary public health threat in the early 1900s, killing nearly 185 of every 100,000 Americans. Better living conditions and medical care caused the rate to drop sharply in the following decades, and it has been on the decline ever since—in fact, almost eradicated. However, beginning in the early 1990s the incidence of tuberculosis has been increasing by 10 to 20 percent each year. The National Institutes of Health attribute the rise to large numbers of AIDS patients, increasing numbers of homeless people, the aging of the U.S. population, and the influx of immigrants from Asian and African countries where TB is largely uncontrolled.

Arthur Schlesinger, Jr., a noted historian and adviser to President Kennedy, often mentioned that American history tends to repeat itself in thirty-year cycles. In 1964, the Surgeon General, Dr. Luther Terry, officially declared cigarettes to be a health hazard. It has taken almost three decades for his warning to be heeded. Cigarettes are being banned from most public places, and we are finally beginning to see an appreciable decline in the total number of smokers. But in 1990 the Centers for Disease Control and Prevention counted more than 400,000 deaths in the United States that were directly attributed to cigarette smoking, not counting cigars, pipes, and smokeless tobacco. That amounted to 20 percent of all deaths in the nation that year—more than from alcohol, drugs, car crashes, and AIDS combined.

Today, in the mid-1990s, we are confronted with an equally ominous threat. As a society, with almost every breath we take, we are "smoking" polluted air. In this chapter, I have documented the dramatic increase of our most common chronic respiratory diseases. Deaths from chronic lung disease—asthma, chronic bronchitis, emphysema—are on the rise. Tuberculosis, a leading killer at the beginning of this century, is making a comeback. More than 92 million Americans, 35 percent, are suffering with a chronic respiratory ailment. Chronic sinusitis and allergic rhinitis have reached epidemic proportions, and our noses and sinuses are failing to protect our lungs. The human respiratory tract is being deluged with a sea of deadly pollutants that relentlessly and insidiously assault our mucous membranes and poison our bodies. The health effects of this modern-day plague may soon prove to be far more devastating than that of cigarettes. But do we have the luxury of waiting another thirty years before responding to the warning? I think not. The crisis is already upon us.

Chapter 5

THE CONVENTIONAL MEDICAL TREATMENT OF SINUSITIS, ASTHMA, ALLERGIES, AND BRONCHITIS

In medical school, doctors are taught to diagnose and treat disease. They learn that body and mind are separate and distinct compartments of a human being, with little interaction between the two. They are trained to focus their attention almost exclusively on the body, and they do so in militaristic terms. They think of the immune system as a defense force on constant alert to protect the body against invasion by bacteria, viruses, allergens, and cancer cells; but they are in a quandary as to how the immune system can be weakened enough to allow infection, allergy, and cancer to occur. Consequently, conventional medicine plays only a reactive role in treating the body: a specific symptom appears and the doctor prescribes drugs or surgery to vanquish or treat it.

What does it mean to treat an ailment? This usually depends on what the condition is. In some instances, treatment implies a cure, with the expectation that the problem will not recur. These treatments are most often surgical. For example, appendicitis is treated with an appendectomy.

At other times, to treat means to relieve symptoms of a chronic condition that has no known cure. These conditions range from cancer and AIDS to the common cold and sore throat. They also include chronic sinusitis, allergic rhinitis, chronic bronchitis, and asthma. Relief of symptoms constitutes the bulk of a physician's work; almost 75 percent of all ailments fall into this treatment realm.

ACUTE AND CHRONIC SINUSITIS

The treatment of acute sinusitis is in yet another category. Acute sinusitis is a bacterial infection in one or more of the sinus cavities. The goal of treatment is to kill the bacteria, open the blocked sinus duct, and restore the mucus-and-cilia cleansing system, while relieving symptoms. Acute sinusitis does have a cure, but the chances of its recurring at some point, either months or years later, are very high.

Acute sinusitis is not a simple infection to treat. Doctors seldom identify the bacteria that cause the infection, so they select an antibiotic to combat the bacteria most likely to have caused the infection. The antibiotic is taken by mouth and absorbed into the bloodstream. Because of the relatively poor blood supply in the sinuses, it usually takes several days before the effect of the drug is felt, especially in adults. Strong antibiotics in relatively high dosages taken for long periods of time are often required.

The next objective is to open the blocked sinus duct and the ostium so that the infected mucus can drain from the sinus. A decongestant opens the duct by shrinking the swollen mucous membrane. However, most decongestants have a drying effect, especially if used in combination with an antihistamine, probably because most commercial decongestants also contain an antihistamine. This drying will thicken the mucus and *prevent* it from draining.

Acute sinusitis is an infection without an accepted standard treatment program. Antibiotics have been, and continue to be, the primary component of the conventional medical treatment. However, if there was one drug that always worked for everyone, this would be a very brief discussion, and I would not have to devote most of the chapter to the subject. The reality is that the efficacy of treatment varies with each patient and with the physician who is administering the treatment. During the past decade, physicians have had to employ greater creativity, using a vastly expanded arsenal of antibiotics, decongestants, expectorants, nasal sprays, and antitussives (cough suppressants) to succeed in treating sinus infections.

Antibiotics

The bacteria most often responsible for causing sinus infections in both adults and children are *Streptococcus pneumoniae* and *Hemophilus influenzae.* Doctors have recently found a marked increase in the incidence of *Staphylococcus aureus,* especially in cases of chronic sinusitis in children, perhaps because of improved diagnostic techniques.

Nasal endoscopy is a procedure usually performed by allergists and ENT physicians using a rod lens telescope that is inserted into the nasal cavity. It permits superior visualization of the interior of the nose, including the opening of ostia, currently being referred to by physicians as the ostio-meatal complex. Intranasal endoscopy can be performed in an office setting using only topical anesthesia, and is easily tolerated by the unsedated patient. It can identify pathologic changes, assist in making the diagnosis of sinusitis, and help to obtain samples of pus for culture. This is a much more accurate method for identifying the bacteria causing the sinus infection than the random nasal swabs that were used in the past. The procedure is also useful for monitoring patient response to medical therapy and for assessing the need for subsequent therapy. Most ENT doctors consider the widespread use of diagnostic nasal endoscopy the greatest single recent advance in sinusitis management.

The physicians who treat the vast majority of patients with acute sinusitis are primary care doctors—family practitioners, internists, and pediatricians, most of whom do not perform nasal endoscopy.

Unfortunately, the antibiotics that effectively treat all the bacteria that cause sinusitis are quite expensive. As sinus infections become more difficult to treat, especially those caused by *Staphylococcus aureus,* researchers have come to the rescue with ever more powerful antibiotics.

For the past decade the drug of choice has been amoxicillin, unless there is an allergy to penicillin. The usual dosage is either 250 or 500 mg (125 or 250 mg in children) three times a day. Both are taken for ten days. This is a routine first step, but it is a hefty dose of antibiotic! Adult patients are told that they should notice definite improvement, with the yellow mucus beginning to clear, in about four to five days. In children the response is usually faster, with fever, nasal drainage, and cough markedly reduced after about forty-eight hours. Patients are instructed to take the medicine for the entire ten days. If this instruction is not followed, the infection often remains. Many physicians routinely prescribe amoxicillin for fourteen days, instead of ten, to reduce the number of treatment failures. For the majority of patients with acute sinusitis, a ten-day course of amoxicillin is all they will need.

In spite of their compliance with instructions, at least 10 percent of patients will call or return to the office shortly after the tenth day, still complaining of most of their symptoms. Some will report that they felt much better while on the antibiotic, but that as soon as they stopped taking it the symptoms recurred. Others will say they experienced no improvement whatsoever.

With the second attempt at treatment, a different antibiotic is selected. The second-choice antibiotics have a bit broader spectrum of efficacy than amoxicillin; all are much more expensive. Table 5-1 lists the second-step drugs that are commonly used for the treatment of sinus infections.

A small but growing percentage of patients are still not cured following a ten-day course of a second-step antibiotic, or their infection returns again shortly after they finish. It sometimes helps to take a two- or even three-week course of the antibiotic and gradually taper it off over the last five to seven days. This seems to allow the body's immune system a better chance to take over for the antibiotic. Whatever the reason, this strategy does

Table 5-1

Second-Step Antibiotics for Sinus Infections —after Amoxicillin

Best drugs for killing both **Streptococcus pneumoniae** *and* **Hemophilus influenzae** *(listed in order of efficacy; those on the same line are roughly equivalent):*
Augmentin
Ceclor, Ceftin, Lorabid
Biaxin
Bactrim, Septra, Cotrim
Vibramycin, Vibra-Tabs (not for children under 8)
Vantin

Best for killing **Staphylococci:**
Augmentin
Ceclor, Ceftin, Lorabid
Duricef, Ultracef, Keflex, Cefanex, Anspor, Velosef
Bactrim, Septra

appear to be more effective than abruptly stopping the drug a patient has been taking for two to three weeks.

Patients who do not respond to antibiotics are good candidates for further diagnostic evaluation with an X-ray, CT scan, or nasal endoscopy to see if there is a physical obstruction of the sinus.

During the past eight years, I have worked with several hundred patients suffering from chronic sinusitis both locally and from thirty different states. I have spoken to a multitude of people, and received many letters from others, who have severe sinusitis. Their stories are striking in their similarity. Almost every one of them had taken multiple antibiotics for their infections, some continuously for a year or more, and yet they were still sick. Many had already undergone sinus surgery, while others had it recommended to them by their physicians.

Antibiotics have been and continue to be the foundation of conventional medical treatment for a sinus infection. But, at this point, I prescribe these drugs only to patients who have one or two sinus infections per year, and have not been taking antibiotics for other reasons. As you will soon learn, they are not absolutely necessary in treating sinus infections. I'm convinced that *the overuse of antibiotics in treating acute sinusitis has become one of the three primary causes of the epidemic of chronic sinusitis.* (The other two are air pollution and emotional stress.)

To be more accurate, I should say the abuse of antibiotics and our dependence upon them in treating a myriad of problems, not just sinus infections, lies at the root of the problem. In recent years, new strains of antibiotic-resistant bacteria, called supergerms, have appeared with a vengeance. According to the Centers for Disease Control and Prevention, 19,000 hospital patients die annually from antibiotic-resistant infections, and another 58,000 people die because of complications attributable to bacterial infections. Many of the people suffering from chronic sinusitis are still sick because their sinuses are infected with antibiotic-resistant bacteria.

Stuart B. Levy, M.D., professor of Medicine, Molecular Biology, and Microbiology; and director of the Center for Adaptation Genetics and Drug Resistance at Tufts University School of Medicine, believes that "up to 50 percent of all antibiotic use in the U.S. today is actually misuse, and some experts estimate that half of all prescriptions written may not even be needed." Dr. Levy is the author of *The Antibiotic Paradox.* The paradox is that the same antibiotics that prevent bacteria from killing people also breed antibiotic-resistant supergerms.

Just as our own species continues to evolve, so do bacteria. They are able to adapt to the attacking antibiotics, and the overuse of these medications provides countless opportunities for bacteria to get to know their enemy and adapt. And it's not just overprescribing by physicians that has created this problem. Most livestock are routinely given antibiotics to fight infections, often in low doses, and milk is allowed to contain eighty different antibiotics. As we ingest antibiotic-laden meat and dairy products, we are contributing to breeding resistant bacteria. Our habit of stopping antibiotic use as soon as symptoms improve also allows resistant strains to survive and flourish.

There is growing evidence that antibiotics interfere with the body's own immune system, hence weakening our ability to fight off the offending bacteria. What may eventually prove to be the most damaging aspect of all in taking antibiotics is that they destroy the friendly bacteria in our digestive tract, which allows for the overgrowth of candida organisms. The subsequent infection of the sinuses by candida has become a primary focus of the Sinus Survival Program in treating chronic sinusitis. This subject will be discussed in depth in Chapter 9.

If you believe you must have antibiotics in order to overcome your infection, then take them for the duration (usually ten days) in order to wipe out all of the pathogenic bacteria. In addition, take acidophilus powder or capsules to replenish the good bacteria in the intestine. There are a number of recommendations in Chapter 9 and throughout Part II that will allow you to strengthen your immune system while you're taking an antibiotic, and when you are not. *Beyond Antibiotics,* by Drs. Michael A. Schmidt, Lendon H. Smith, and Keith W. Sehnert is an excellent reference book on this subject.

Decongestants and Expectorants

The decongestants are specifically used to open the ostia and sinus ducts while relieving the symptoms of head and nasal congestion, headache, facial pain, and, to some extent, sore throat and cough. Expectorants, which are mucus thinners, can help to relieve the same symptoms.

The challenge of using a decongestant is to find one whose benefits outweigh its side effects. Decongestants are readily available in many familiar over-the-counter (OTC) products, such as Dristan, Contac, Allerest, Drixoral, Actifed, Dimetapp, Triaminicin, and a host of other cold remedies. Every one of these contains an antihistamine in combination with the decongestant. This is also true of Sinutab and many other sinus reme-

Table 5-2

Decongestants with Analgesics (OTC)

Advil Cold and Sinus Caplets
Allerest No Drowsiness Tablets
Bayer Select Maximum Strength Sinus Pain Relief Caplets
Congesprin Cold Tablets for Children
Contact Non-Drowsy Formula Sinus Caplets
Dimetapp Sinus Caplets
Dristan Cold Caplets
Dristan Maximum Strength Caplets
Dristan Sinus Tablets
Maximum Strength Ornex Caplets
Ornex Caplets
Sinarest No Drowsiness Tablets
Sine-Aid Maximum Strength Caplets, Gelcaps, and Tablets
Sine-Off Maximum Strength No Drowsiness Formula Caplets
Sinus Excedrin Extra Strength Tablets and Caplets
Sinutab Maximum Strength Without Drowsiness Caplets and
  Tablets
Sudafed Maximum Strength Sinus Tablets and Caplets
Tylenol Maximum Strength Sinus Tablets, Caplets, and Gelcaps

dies. Given the drying effect of antihistamines and the subsequent thickening of the mucus, I am convinced they do more harm than good. They are fine if all you are trying to treat is a cold, but I believe that in many instances they have actually helped a cold progress into a sinus infection. If you have a history of sinus problems, I would advise you to avoid antihistamines. If you are not sure about the ingredients of an OTC product, ask a pharmacist.

The most common ingredients in both prescription and OTC decongestants are pseudoephedrine, phenylpropanolamine, and phenylephrine. Each works in much the same way to shrink swollen mucous membranes and reduce nasal and sinus congestion. Many products contain these decongestants in combination. Some, available only by prescription, include two of these ingredients; others only one, along with a pain reliever or an expectorant or cough suppressant.

There is a myriad of choices at the pharmacy. The following is a guide to lead you through the confusing maze of cold and sinus preparations. Before you begin the process, it would be helpful to ask yourself what it is you are treating. What are the symptoms that most trouble you? Are you stuffed up? Or is it the headache, the cough, the sore throat, or the thick mucus that you would most like to eliminate? Since you probably have more than one symptom, you will be looking for a decongestant in combination with something else. However, choose anything but an antihistamine. I recommend the preparations in tables 5-2 through 5-6. If all you need is a plain decongestant, then Sudafed tablets are an excellent choice. If you have a lot of thick mucus draining, don't want a decongestant, and would like a simple expectorant, Fenesin, Humibid, and Organidin are all good prescription drugs.

Tables 5-2, 5-3, and 5-6 all list OTC products. Please follow the dosage instructions on the bottle or package. The drugs in Table 5-4, which your doctor might prescribe, contain the same decongestants and expectorants as those found in the OTC products. The primary difference is that these drugs contain higher doses and are long-acting, continuing to work for up to twelve hours. The exceptions are Entex and Dura-Gest capsules, the latter of which is both a brand-name drug and used by most pharmacists as the generic form of Entex. These short-acting products can be taken every four to six hours and contain two decongestants, phenylephrine and phenylpropanolamine, in combination with the expectorant guaifenesin. I find them more effective in the treatment of acute sinusitis than the long-acting preparations. Avoid them if you have high blood pressure. They can cause insomnia in adults, but some young children experience the opposite side effect and become drowsy. Omitting the bedtime dose usually eliminates the insomnia.

I usually don't encourage patients to take the decongestant on the same rigid schedule as the antibiotic, or for the entire ten-day course. I tell them to take it regularly for the first four to five

Table 5-3

Decongestants with Expectorants (OTC)

Glycofed Tablets
Guaitab Tablets
Naldecon Ex Pediatric Drops
Robitussin-PE Syrup
Triaminic Expectorant

Table 5-4

Decongestants with Expectorants (Rx)

Deconasal II Tablets
Deconasal Sprinkle Capsules
Dura-Gest Capsules
Dura-Vent Tablets
Endal Tablets
Entex Capsules
Entex LA Tablets
Entex Liquid
Guaifed Capsules
Guaifed-PD Capsules
Nolex LA Tablets
Respaire-60 Capsules
Respaire-120 Capsules
Ru-Tuss DE Tablets
Sinupan Capsules
Zephrex Tablets
Zephrex LA Tablets

days, then gradually taper off. If they still experience head and sinus congestion, they should continue the ten-day course. Patients with active sinus infections should avoid air travel because of the pressure changes and poor air quality found on airplanes. If they can't, I recommend taking a decongestant approximately two hours prior to the scheduled landing.

Decongestant Sprays

An OTC alternative for those with extreme head and nasal congestion or sinus pain is nasal decongestant spray. There are several twelve-hour varieties from which to choose, including Afrin, Dristan, Sinex, Neo-Synephrine, and Vicks. These should be used with great caution and only for two or three days at most. They can easily become addictive! They produce what is called a rebound effect, which means that as their decongestant effect wears off and the head and nasal congestion return, the feeling of stuffiness is worse than it was before using the spray. This elicits a strong desire to spray again, and a vicious cycle begins. Be careful!

If you have been using a spray regularly and are unable to stop, you probably need some help. Consult with your physician and tell him honestly what has been happening. I have had a high success rate helping patients to break this habit with the following regimen:

- Throw away the nasal spray.
- Take a tapered dose of cortisone over a one-week period, either Medrol (the generic name is methylprednisolone) in the 4-mg dosepak or 5 mg of prednisone. These are prescription drugs that relieve inflammation.
- Take forty capsules of Entex or Dura-Gest in a tapered schedule: one capsule three times a day over seven days; then one capsule two times a day over seven days; followed by one capsule daily before bed over seven days.
- Use moisture—including saline nasal spray, a humidifier, and steaming in the bathroom (refer to this chapter's Moisture and Irrigation section)—and one or more of the natural decongestants listed under "Stuffy Nose" in Table 8-3, p. 173, "Natural Quick-Fix Symptom Treatment."

Remember that it is extremely difficult to keep your sinuses healthy with *continued* use of a decongestant nasal spray. However, one instance in which it can be quite helpful is during air travel. If you have a stuffy nose before embarking on your trip, plan to use the spray shortly before you begin the descent.

Antitussives (Cough Suppressants)

If a patient's chief complaint is a cough that interrupts sleep, I will withhold the bedtime dose of decongestant and substitute a strong prescription cough suppressant containing either codeine or hydrocodone in combination with a decongestant, an expectorant, or both. Such antitussives can cause drowsiness, which is why I rarely recommend them for daytime use. Besides, these people are already tired from having a sinus infection. They don't need any additional sedation. The most commonly prescribed antitussives for sinus patients are listed in Table 5-5. If a cough suppressant is indicated for use during the day, especially in children, there are several similar OTC combination drugs from which to choose. They can be taken by both adults and children. The most commonly used and easily found are listed in Table 5-6.

Analgesics (Pain Relievers)

To relieve the frequent symptoms of headache, facial pain, and sore throat, I recommend the OTC pain relievers Advil and Nuprin. Both contain ibuprofen, which not only relieves pain but reduces inflammation. (To some extent, ibuprofen also can lower a fever.) Both pain relievers are dispensed in 200-mg tablets, and they are safe for *adults* in dosages of three or even four at a time if the pain is especially severe. This high dosage, however, should be taken with food, especially if there is a history of stomach ulcers. Since the headache is usually accompanied by some degree of nasal and/or head congestion, the Advil Cold and Sinus Caplets are an effective and recent option available to sinus sufferers.

Table 5-5

Antitussives with Decongestants or Expectorants (Rx)*

Donatussin DC Syrup
Humibid DM Tablets and Sprinkle Capsules
Hycomine Pediatric Syrup
Hycomine Syrup
Naldecon CX Liquid
Novahistine Expectorant Liquid
Nucofed Expectorant Syrup
Nucofed Syrup
Nucofed Pediatric Expectorant Syrup
Robitussin A-C
Robitussin-DAC
Triaminic Expectorant with Codeine
Tussi Organidin
Tussi Organidin DM

* Check with your pharmacist for updated changes in these products.

   Aspirin has the same effects as ibuprofen but doesn't seem to be as strong. Tylenol and other acetaminophen–containing products are simply analgesics, with no effect on the inflamed sinuses. However, if lowering a fever is the primary objective, both aspirin and Tylenol would be better choices. Any acetaminophen-containing product is the drug of choice for children with acute sinusitis.

Moisture and Irrigation

Moisture helps empty the sinus of its thick, infected mucus, and in doing so helps restore normal cilial function and relieves nasal and head congestion, headache, sinus pain, and sore throat. Warm, moist air is best, and the easiest place to get it is in the bathroom. Steamers can now be installed in showers, or simply

Table 5-6

Antitussives with Decongestants and Expectorants (OTC)

Benylin Expectorant Liquid★
Cheracol D Cough Liquid★
Comtrex Cough Formula
Contac Cough and Chest and Cold Liquid
Diamacol Caplets
Dorcol Children's Cough Syrup
Formula 44D Decongestant Cough Mixture
Formula 44M Liquid
Naldecon DX Pediatric Drops
Naldecon DX Children's Syrup
Naldecon DX Adult Liquid
Naldecon Senior DX Liquid★
Novahistine DXM Liquid
Robitussin-CF Liquid
Robitussin DM Cough Calmers Lozenges★
Robitussin DM Syrup★
Ru-Tuss Expectorant Liquid
Sudafed Cough Syrup
Sudafed Cold and Cough Liquid Caps
Vicks Day Quil Caps and Liquid

★ Contains no decongestant.

close any doors and windows and turn the shower on hot to create steam. You then have the choice of either getting in the shower, after adjusting the temperature, of course, or just sitting and relaxing in the steam until you run out of hot water. Make a conscious effort to breathe through your nose. Hot towels applied over the face can also be helpful.

As most of us do not have an endless supply of hot water or steamers, making a steam room of the bathroom can be done only two or three times a day. What about the rest of the time? If you are staying home from work, your best source of moist air is a humidifier placed by your bed, with the bedroom door and windows closed. Most humidifiers are quiet and very effective in producing a moist environment in an enclosed space. They are available in pharmacies, department stores, and hardware stores under a variety of brand names. The one I know best and with which I have enjoyed excellent results is the Bionaire-Clear Mist 5 (CMP-5). Although the ideal humidifier has probably not yet been designed, this one comes as close I've been able to find. It quietly yet powerfully puts out warm moisture, can cover an area of up to 1,600 square feet, and is relatively easy to clean. The Kenmore Warm Mist is the identical unit, and it is available at most Sears stores. These units cost about $125.

The cool-mist ultrasonics put out a fine mineral dust unless distilled water is used to fill them, and the new warm ultrasonics have a tendency to break down. Steam humidifiers or vaporizers can become quite hot, which could be a concern if you have small children. The ultrasonic humidifiers with a demineralizing component seem to have eliminated most problems. Whatever your choice, be sure the reservoir tank opening is large enough to allow for cleaning. Wipe and cleanse the tank at least weekly with vinegar water; otherwise it becomes a breeding ground for molds. During treatment for a sinus infection, the humidifier should be used every night while you sleep. It's also a good idea to fill it and turn it on as soon as you come home from work so your bedroom will be warm and moist (and cozy) by the time you're ready for bed. The moisture is very helpful in relieving the infection's cough and sore throat during the night.

Another device I've been using preventively on myself and recommending to patients as part of their treatment program is the Steam Inhaler (see Figure 5-1). It's extremely effective for thinning and loosening the thick infected mucus stuck in the sinuses, and can also be quite soothing to dry and irritated mucous membranes. A drop of eucalyptus oil added to the unit while you are steaming enhances its beneficial effect. It works extremely well as a nasal decongestant and for relieving sinus headaches. If used just prior to nasal irrigation, a procedure that I'm about to explain, it will greatly increase the benefit of the irrigation. The Steam Inhaler costs about $40 and is available in

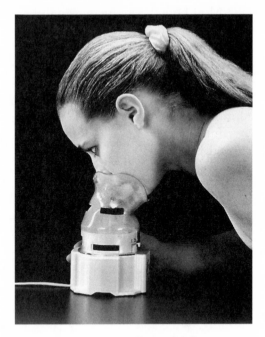

FIGURE 5-1.　*Steam Inhaler*

some pharmacies. Complete information on where to obtain any of the products I mention is listed in the Product Index at the end of the book.

Far more expensive than the Steam Inhaler, but also more effective as a nasal decongestant and in helping the sinuses to drain, is the Rhinotherm® unit. This device has had limited availability for the past four years and is familiar to a small but growing number of ENT physicians. Based on the principle of hyperthermia, Rhinotherm delivers 100 percent water-saturated pressurized air, at a temperature of 110°F, directly into the nasal passages. A microprocessor controls the ultrasonic transducer, which vibrates the water into droplets of approximately 4 to 8 microns. The heated water is then mixed with air, and administered to both nostrils via a hand-held tube.

Relief from nasal congestion after a Rhinotherm treatment can last, on average, for three and a half days. However, with sinus infections, I recommend treatments (lasting fifteen to thirty minutes) two or three times a day.

Assuming your environment is relatively dry, as indoor air tends to be during the winter months in most parts of the United States, you can provide moisture with a saltwater, also called saline, nasal spray. There are several commercial products available in pharmacies. However, you can make your own saline spray by mixing $1/3$ teaspoon of non-iodized table salt and a pinch of baking soda in an 8-ounce cup of lukewarm bottled water (without chlorine) and dispensing it from a spray bottle. Do not use sea salt (it has iodine). Spray into each nostril while closing off the other nostril and simultaneously inhaling. This is nonaddictive and can be done as often as you like throughout the day. It has no negative side effects, except for the curious looks you will get from those wanting to know what in the world you are doing.

In recent years, I have been testing an exciting product that I have formulated and developed with Dr. Steve Morris, a naturopathic physician from Seattle. The Sinus Survival Spray consists mostly of saline along with very small amounts of several herbs. It will soon be available in many health food stores. I will discuss its ingredients and benefits in Chapter 8 since this chapter presents a comprehensive but "conventional" medical treatment plan. This section, "Moisture and Irrigation," and the following, "Hydration and Bed Rest," are actually the only aspects of the conventional approach that are also an integral part of the holistic medical treatment for chronic sinusitis to be presented in Part II.

An even more effective way of moisturizing is saline irrigation. This procedure can result in dramatic relief from pain, in that it reduces swelling in the nasal passages, causing a reduction of pressure in the sinus, as well as helping to empty the sinus of its infected mucus. Saltwater sprays also irrigate: i.e., wash out some mucus, bacteria, and dust particles, while reducing swelling. However, they don't do it as well as the following irrigation methods, which should be done three to four times a day, for acute sinusitis and once or twice with a milder chronic condition.

Mix the saline solution for irrigation fresh each day in one cup of lukewarm bottled water. Add $1/3$ teaspoon of non–iodized table salt and a tiny pinch of baking soda, thus making the solution close to normal body fluid salinity and pH. Irrigating with plain water is usually somewhat uncomfortable. Use the full cup of saline solution for each irrigation (one-half cup for each nostril), irrigating over the sink, with the head in an upright position, using one of the following methods, but in an upright position. Always blow your nose *very* gently after irrigating.

Method 1: Completely fill a large, all–rubber ear syringe (available at most pharmacies) with saline solution. Lean over the sink, pinch one nostril closed, and insert the syringe tip just inside the open nostril, pinching the nostril around the tip. *Gently* squeeze and release the bulb several times to swish the solution around the inside of your nose. The solution will run out both nostrils and might also run out of your mouth. Repeat this for each nostril until one cup of saline solution is used, or until the solution is clear.

Method 2: Pour saline solution into the palm of your hand and sniff the solution up your nose, one nostril at a time.

Method 3: Use an angled nasal irrigator attachment (the Grossan nasal irrigator is available at some pharmacies) on a Water Pik appliance. Set the Water Pik at the lowest possible pressure and insert the irrigator tip just inside one nostril, pinching your nostril to form a seal. Irrigate with your mouth open, allowing the fluid to drain out either your mouth or nose. Repeat the procedure in the other nostril.

Method 4: For very small children, irrigate with ten to twenty drops of saline solution per nostril from an eyedropper.

Method 5: For the past two years I have been recommending the use of the Neti Pot for nasal irrigation (see Figure 5-2). A small porcelain pot with a narrow spout, it works in much the same way as the ear syringe and the Grossan nasal irrigator, but more gently and conveniently. Because of this, people with

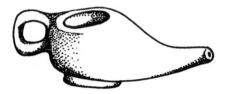

FIGURE 5-2.   *Neti Pot*

chronic sinusitis are much more apt to use this method on a regular basis, both therapeutically in treating an infection and preventively. Of all the treatment options suggested in this book for curing chronic sinusitis, nasal irrigation is probably one of the most helpful. The Neti Pot is made by the Himalayan Institute in Honesdale, Pennsylvania, and is available in many health food stores.

If you are using a decongestant nasal spray, use it only *after* the saltwater nasal irrigations.

These methods obviously require more effort than the saline nasal sprays, but many patients comment on how much more helpful it is.

Another solution that has been effective in irrigation is called Alkalol. It is a mucus solvent and cleaner, and can be used with the saline solution in a 1:1 ratio ($^{1}/_{2}$ saline, $^{1}/_{2}$ Alkalol) with all of the methods previously mentioned. You will probably have to ask your pharmacist to order it for you, as it is not usually available, but Alkalol is very inexpensive.

Moisture, saline spray, and irrigation can also help to relieve the symptoms of dry, crusted nasal membranes that are common with chronic sinusitis and often prone to nosebleeds. You can apply Neosporin ointment or Ponaris nasal emollient to the nasal membranes twice daily with a Q-tip or your little finger.

Hydration and Bed Rest

In regard to a cold, you have often heard the advice to drink a lot of liquids and stay in bed. For acute sinusitis, this advice is good. I recommend at least eight to ten 8-ounce glasses of water daily. Avoid ice-cold drinks and anything containing caffeine, sugar, or alcohol.

As for resting, try to listen to your body and not push yourself. As a general rule, if you are waking up to an alarm clock you are not getting enough sleep. Allow your body to tell you how much sleep you need and adjust your bedtime accordingly. Rest as much as possible during the first five to seven days of treatment.

Sinus Surgery

If you have completed several courses of antibiotics, have strictly adhered to all of your primary care physician's recommendations, and you are still infected, your next step is often a referral to an ear, nose, and throat specialist. Otolaryngologists are the professionals usually assigned the task of treating the most challenging chronic sinus sufferers—group 1—described in Chapter 3. The sinus patients in this group suffer the most discomfort. Before arriving at the specialist's office, they might have been fighting a sinus infection for several months to a year, and in many cases, two or three years. Most of them have already been through multiple courses of antibiotics without success. Their physicians have given up; these patients are considered treatment failures.

The initial evaluation by the ENT doctor usually includes the application of a topical decongestant in the nose and a nasal bacterial culture, followed by a physical examination of the nose, throat, and sinuses. The specimen for the culture is usually obtained using nasal endoscopy and needs to be obtained right from the opening of the sinus ducts (ostia) or else it will be of little value. The ENT specialist is attempting to identify the specific bacteria that are infecting the sinuses. The bacteria found in the nose are not usually the same as those infecting the sinuses. The culture should be performed by someone who has had a lot of experience with endoscopy and in locating the ostia so that the results will be a true reflection of the bacteria that are actually causing the infection. This test is critical to the selection of the most effective antibiotic. As a result of the more accurate performance of this test, many specialists have seen a dramatic increase in *Staphylococcus aureus* in the sinuses. This has been one of the most difficult bacteria to treat.

Subsequent diagnostic procedures might include a sinus CT scan to determine if, after a course of an antibiotic, there are any lingering pockets of infection; nasal endoscopy, to see if there is any obstruction around the ostia; a nasal cytogram, a microscopic inspection of cells from the nasal mucous membrane; and a complete battery of skin and/or blood tests to identify possible allergies.

The initial treatment usually includes a ten-day to two-week course of one of the second-step antibiotics (see Table 5-1) —in addition to the treatment regimen that has just been described in this chapter, with particular emphasis on irrigation. If this fails—meaning either that there is no improvement or that the infection is still present on the CT scan or recurs shortly after the antibiotic is stopped—further evaluation using one or more of the diagnostic procedures previously mentioned will be necessary. Depending on the results, either a different antibiotic or surgery will be offered.

Sinus surgery has improved dramatically over the past decade. If there is an obstruction of the ostio-meatal complex (the opening of the sinus duct into the nasal passage), surgery is usually recommended. The endoscope has taken sinus surgery to an even higher level of success. The most common endoscopic sinus surgery is a bilateral middle antrostomy, in which the maxillary sinus ostia are enlarged from 2 millimeters to about 10 or 12 millimeters (approximately the width of a dime). This procedure is a marked improvement over the surgery that created naso-antral windows—the most common procedure prior to endoscopic surgery. The opening of a naso-antral window was about the same size as the opening created by an antrostomy, but it went entirely through the bony medial wall (nasal side) of the maxillary sinus. The new procedure is not only less destructive, but preserves the normal direction of mucus flow in the sinus. Mucus naturally flows out through the sinus duct and into the nose. The fact that the naso–antral window was not in the best position to enhance drainage greatly diminished its rate of success, despite the large opening it produced. Many patients who have had this surgery, or the Caldwell-Luc operation or ethmoidectomy (other surgical procedures not performed as often anymore), continue to have sinus problems and not infrequently require additional surgery.

Endoscopic surgery has been widely performed since 1988 and it is clearly an improvement over the previous procedures. It is performed on an outpatient basis under local anesthesia, and patients can expect to miss only about one week of work. It is certainly not inexpensive, with surgeons charging anywhere from $3,000 to $10,000 for the procedure. However, it is still a long way from a guaranteed cure for chronic sinusitis. What I am observing with increasing frequency is that many people experience short-term improvement, six months to one year, and then begin the cycle of sinus infections and antibiotics over again. One difference seems to be that they are not as uncomfortable with their infections as they were prior to surgery. This is probably because their sinuses are able to drain more easily. Other people I've treated have seen no change in their condition following this surgery.

In spite of technological and therapeutic advances, sinus surgery has been and will continue to be most successful in those instances in which it eliminates one or more of the obstructive causes of sinusitis, such as polyps, cysts, an enlarged or distorted nasal turbinate (turbinate hypertrophy), and a deviated septum. But even in these cases, the surgery is still treating the symptom, not the cause. What is responsible for stimulating the growth of the polyps, cysts, and swollen turbinates in nasal mucous membranes to such an extent that a congenital deviated septum is now all of a sudden obstructing the sinus from draining? Most ENT surgeons claim that there is no known cause for these phenomena. They just happen. Many patients who have had polyps surgically removed have seen them recur. And what about the other surgical cases of chronic sinusitis that do not involve one of these obstructive causes? Have all therapeutic options been tried prior to the decision to have surgery? In most cases, they have not, because all of the physical, environmental, emotional, mental, social, and spiritual factors that contribute to sinus disease have not been addressed. Until they are incorporated into the therapeutic approach, the conventional medical treatment for chronic sinusitis will continue as a symptom-focused regimen, and chronic sinusitis will remain a largely incurable problem with the prognosis "You're going to have to learn to live with it."

For the most part, the conventional medical treatment for the other respiratory diseases is also based on relieving symptoms with medication. Unlike sinusitis, there is no "last resort" surgical procedure available if "all else fails."

ASTHMA

According to the NIH "Guidelines for the Diagnosis and Management of Asthma," effective management of asthma relies on four integral components:

- objective measures of lung function, not only to assess but also to monitor each patient's asthma;
- pharmacologic therapy;
- environmental measures to control allergens and irritants;
- patient education.

Effective management of asthma has the following goals:

- to maintain (near) "normal" pulmonary function rates;
- to maintain normal activity levels (including exercise);
- to prevent chronic and troublesome symptoms (e.g., coughing or breathlessness in the night, in the early morning, or after exertion);

- to prevent recurrent exacerbations (flare-ups) of asthma;
- to avoid adverse effects from asthma medications.

Although patient education, environmental measures, and pulmonary function tests are all an integral part of the treatment program, the attainment of these goals for managing chronic asthma relies heavily on the proper administration of pharmaceutical drugs. The treatment of an acute asthma attack, often considered a medical emergency, is totally dependent upon medication. Conventional medicine frequently performs "miracles" for these patients, who are unable to breathe and are confronting death by suffocation. In these critical situations, the conventional approach is clearly superior to anything else.

Notice, however, that the objective in treating chronic asthma is "management." There is no mention of *curing* this disease. The general principles involved in managing chronic asthma include:

- Treat the underlying pathology of asthma. First-line therapy should focus on preventing or reversing the airway inflammation that is a principal factor in the airway hyperresponsiveness that characterizes asthma and determines symptoms, disease severity, and possibly mortality.
- Tailor general therapy guidelines to individual needs. Specific asthma therapy, dictated by the severity of the disease, medication tolerance, and sensitivity to environmental allergens, must be selected to fit the needs of individual patients.
- Treat asthma triggers, associated conditions, and special problems: exposure to known allergens and irritants must be reduced or eliminated; colds, sinus infections, middle ear infections (otitis media), and allergic rhinitis can set off or aggravate asthma. Treatment of a known trigger prior to exposure, such as exercise, is recommended. Influenza vaccinations and pneumococcal vaccines should be considered for patients with moderate or severe asthma.
- Seek consultation with an asthma specialist for pulmonary function studies, evaluation of the role of allergy and irritants,

or evaluation of the medication plan if the goals of therapy are not achieved.

- Use step-care pharmacologic therapy. An aim of this therapy is to use the optimum medication needed to maintain control with minimal risk for adverse effects. The step-care approach, in which the number of medications and frequency of administration are increased as necessary, is used to achieve this aim.
- Monitor continually. Continual monitoring, including pulmonary function tests and regular visits to your physician, are necessary to assure that therapeutic goals are met.

The medications include:
- *Anti-inflammatory agents:* They interrupt the development of bronchial inflammation and have a preventive action. They also mitigate ongoing inflammatory reactions in the airways. These drugs include corticosteroids, cromolyn sodium or cromolyn-like compounds. *Oral corticosteroids,* such as prednisone, prednisolone, or medrol, are often used in the early treatment of severe acute asthma attacks to prevent their progression, to reduce the need for emergency room visits or hospitalizations, and to reduce the severity of the disease. When they're used to treat acute asthma, the onset of action occurs approximately three hours after administration, with peak effectiveness occurring after six to twelve hours. Oral or intravenous corticosteroids are associated with many adverse effects in both short- and long-term use. Short-term major adverse effects include reversible abnormalities in glucose (sugar) metabolism, increased appetite, fluid retention, weight gain, rounding of the face, mood alteration, hypertension (high blood pressure), and peptic (stomach/duodenal) ulcer. Long-term risks include osteoporosis, hypertension, cataracts, and impaired immune function.

Inhaled corticosteroids are considered safe and are being used as primary therapy for moderate and severe asthma. Their use not only provides symptomatic benefit but also reduces airway hyperresponsiveness. The most frequently prescribed inhaled corticosteroids are Azmacort, Beclovent, AeroBid, Vanceril, and Decadron Phosphate Respihaler.

Administered preventively, cromolyn sodium inhibits allergen-induced airway narrowing as well as acute airway narrowing after exercise and after exposure to cold dry air and sulfur dioxide. The mechanism of action of cromolyn is not fully understood, nor can it be reliably predicted whether or not a patient will respond to it. A four-to-six-week trial therapy is often required to determine its efficacy. Cromolyn sodium is available as Intal in a capsule, powder, or nebulizer solution. It also comes in a tablet called Gastrocrom.

- *Bronchodilators:* These drugs act principally to dilate the airways by relaxing bronchial smooth muscle. They include beta-adrenergic agonists, methylxanthines, and anticholinergics.

    Inhaled beta-adrenergic agonists are the medication of choice for treatment of acute exacerbations of asthma and for the prevention of exercise-induced asthma. They have also been used chronically to aid in the control of persistent airway narrowing, but recent reports suggest prolonged, regular administration (as opposed to as-needed use) of a potent inhaled beta-agonist might result in diminished control of asthma and might even be *a contributing factor in the increasing asthmatic death toll in children.* Therefore, they should be used *only* for acute airway obstruction and not for routine, scheduled therapy. They are best administered via metered dose inhaler or nebulizer. The most frequently prescribed beta-agonist inhalers are Alupent, Brethaire, Bronkometer, Isuprel Mistometer, Maxair, Metaprel, Proventil, Serevent, and Ventolin. Alupent, Metaprel, Proventil, and Ventolin might also be prescribed in the form of tablets or syrup.

    The principal methylxanthine used in asthma therapy is theophylline. Although the precise mechanism for its action is not clear, theophylline serves as a mild-to-moderate bronchodilator depending upon its blood level. When given in a sustained-release preparation, it has a long duration of action and is particularly useful in the control of nocturnal asthma. Theophylline has the potential for significant adverse effects if it exceeds the recommended blood level. Nausea and vomiting are the most common signs of early toxicity. Seizures may occur and children may experience behavioral disturbances. Rapid heart rate (tachycardia), abnormal heart rhythm (arrhythmia), difficult urination in older men, and elevated blood sugar and potassium are other possible side effects. To avoid these problems it is recommended that theophylline blood levels be checked frequently when beginning therapy and at regular intervals of six to twelve months thereafter. There are a number of frequently prescribed methylxanthine medications, most of which contain theophylline. They include: Aerolate, Bronkodyl, Choledyl, Dilor, Elixophyllin, Lufyllin, Marax, Quibron, Respbid, Slo-bid, Slo-Phyllin, Tedral, Theo-Dur, Theo-24, Theolair, and Uniphyl. Most of these are available in both liquid and tablet form. There are also rectal suppositories containing aminophylline, another methylxanthine.

Anticholinergics, such as Atrovent, are bronchodilators that are infrequently used because of the length of time for onset of action and a number of unpleasant side effects.

Primatene Mist and tablets and Sudafed are bronchodilators consistently available over the counter. Sudafed, containing the drug ephedrine, is usually used as a nasal decongestant but also has a bronchodilating effect. Primatene tablets contain both theophylline and ephedrine. They should be used only as needed for acute asthmatic attacks and not on a regular basis. Tedral is also available in some states without a prescription. Besides Primatene Mist, other OTC beta-agonists include AsthmaHaler Mist, Bronitin Mist, Bronkaid Mist, and Medihaler-Epi. They all contain the drug epinephrine bitartrate.

Since there is an abundance of thick mucus found in the airways of asthmatics, it is usually helpful to take an expectorant along with a bronchodilator. Expectorants thin the mucus and make it easier to cough up. It is for this reason that cough suppressants are not recommended for asthmatics. Prescription expectorants containing either guaifenesin or iodinated glycerol include: Fenesin, Humibid, Organidin, Sinumist, and SSKI. There are also a number of OTC products that contain guaifenesin such as Guiatuss, Anti-Tuss, Genatuss, Glyate, Halotussin, Malotuss, Robitussin, Uni-tussin, Naldecon Senior EX, Breonesin, Hytuss 2X, and Glycotuss. Terpin Hydrate is another OTC expectorant.

There are several combination prescription drugs that contain both a bronchodilator (usually theophylline) and an expectorant, and are available in tablets and liquid. Some of these are Quibron-300, Glyceryl T, Slo-Phyllin GG, Asbron G Inlay, Midrane GG-2, Theolate, Theophylline KI, Elixophyllin KI, Dilor-G, Lufyllin-GG, Theo-Organidin, and Brondelate. Two OTC combination drugs that contain theophylline, ephedrine, and guaifenesin are Primatene Dual Action tablets and Bronkaid tablets. Bronkotabs have the same three ingredients plus phenobarbital, and are also OTC.

According to the NIH guidelines, the classification for asthma is as follows:

- mild asthma: Mild, episodic asthma that requires inhaled beta-agonists less than two times per week.
- moderate asthma: Asthma that is not controlled with as-needed use of inhaled beta-agonists. The addition of inhaled corticosteroids, Intal, sustained-release theophyllines, or oral beta-agonists is required.
- severe asthma: Asthma that is not controlled on maximum doses of bronchodilators (oral and inhaled) and an inhaled anti-inflammatory agent.

Not only is asthma classified by its response to drug therapy, but its treatment is largely based upon these powerful medications. Although almost every one of them has the potential for causing seriously adverse side effects, they do allow people with asthma to *manage* their condition and live a somewhat "normal" life. While extremely beneficial, the conventional medical treatment for asthma also creates a drug-dependence and alleviates the need and desire for most asthmatics to address the multiple causes of their disease and subsequently to cure it.

ALLERGIES

The treatment for allergic rhinitis, or hay fever, besides removing the offending allergen, consists of medication and allergy desensitization injections.

Eliminating the allergen is usually a bit of a challenge. Avoiding allergenic foods can be relatively simple, but getting rid of the family pet if you're allergic to cats, or escaping from pollen is much more difficult. One option for allergic cat owners is to wash the cat once a month, and within three to eight months it will stop making the offending allergen in its saliva. You will have created a nonallergenic cat.

You can minimize pollen exposure by taking refuge in sealed, air-conditioned office buildings and houses, where filters cleanse most of the offending pollen from incoming air. For those allergy sufferers unconcerned with domestic decor, the NIH recommends the following steps to achieve a dust-free and dust mite–free bedroom: Remove carpeting, upholstered furniture, heavy curtains, venetian blinds, fuzzy wool blankets, and comforters stuffed with wool or feathers. Empty the room, scrub it and everything that is to be returned to it, and thereafter thoroughly clean the room every week. If replacing curtains, hang some that are lightweight and can be laundered weekly. Replace the comfortable chairs with wooden or metal ones that can be scrubbed, keep clothing in plastic zippered bags and shoes in closed boxes off the floor.

For temporary relief of mild allergies, doctors usually prescribe antihistamines. For years these drugs almost always caused drowsiness, but now there are a few that do not have this inconvenient side effect. Seldane, Hismanal, and Claritin are all non-sedating prescription options. There are a number of OTC antihistamines, either alone or in combination with decongestants. (See

Table 5-7

Decongestant and Antihistamine Combinations OTC

Dallergy-D Capsules
Chlor-Trimeton 12 hour Relief
Chlor-Trimeton 4 hour Relief
Co-Pyronil 2 Pulvules
Fedanist Tablets
Sudafed Plus Tablets
Allerest Maximum Strength
Allerest 12 Hour Caplets
Contac Maximum Strength 12 Hour Caplets
Triaminic-12 Tablets
Triaminic Cold Tablets
Demazin Tablets
Dimetapp Extentabs
Cheracol Sinus Tablets
Drixoral Cold and Allergy Tablets
12 Hour Cold Tabs
Tavist D Tablets
Dristan Allergy Capsules
Dimetane Decongestant Caplets
Benadryl Decongestant Tablets
Actifed Tablets
Allercon Tablets
Allergy Cold Tablets

tables 5-7 and 5-8.) The stimulant effect of the decongestant sometimes counteracts the sedation of the antihistamine. I would recommend trying some of the OTCs before opting for a prescription. The latter are considerably more expensive. Some of the OTC antihistamines containing the drug diphenhydramine are Benadryl-25, AllerMax, Dormarex 2, Banophen, Belix, Genahist, Nidryl, Phendry, Benylin Cough, Hydramine Cough, and generics. There are others that have chlorpheniramine maleate: Chlor-Trimeton, Teldrin, Chlor-Amine, Aller-Chlor, and Chlorate.

Many allergy sufferers also derive significant benefit from the antiallergic and anti-inflammatory effects of the prescription corticosteroid nasal sprays such as Beconase, Vancenase, Nasalide, and Nasacort. Cromolyn sodium has a similar action and is available as a nasal spray (Nasalcrom) and as an eye drop (Opticrom). The effect of the spray seems to be enhanced if used after nasal irrigation. Irrigation removes the mucus secretions so the prescription spray does not sit on the mucus but hits the lining of the nose directly. The irrigation also removes allergens such as pollen and dust. A seasonal pollen allergy sufferer, especially one who is also prone to sinus infections, should use the spray on a maintenance schedule throughout most of the allergy season, about one to two months. Long-term use of these cortisone sprays, beyond three months, can cause chronic irritation, inflammation, and increased mucus secretion. This is less of a problem with the aqueous-based than the Freon-based sprays. The potentially serious side effects that can accompany the oral administration of corticosteroids, such as Prednisone, are not a risk with the sprays since they are very minimally absorbed into the bloodstream.

Table 5-8

Decongestant and Antihistamine SUGAR-FREE OTC

Chlorafed Liquid (alcohol and dye free)
Hayfebrol Liquid (alcohol and dye free)
Ryna Liquid (alcohol and dye free)
Trind Liquid
Novahistine Elixir
Bromanate Elixir
Bromatapp Elixir
Bromphen Elixir
Partapp Elixir

If you are not satisfied with the symptomatic relief you have received from antihistamines and steroid nasal sprays, your next step will often be a visit to an allergist. Depending upon the results of a battery of allergy skin tests, you might then be considered a candidate for allergy desensitization injections. These shots, containing very small amounts of the offending allergen(s), will often be given a few days apart early on, and progress to monthly injections that could last for several years. People with severe pollen allergy seem to benefit most from this course of treatment, while those with mold, dust-mite, and animal dander allergies do not fare as well. Why the shots do and sometimes don't work remains a mystery. Whether or not they do, however, they are consistently an expensive treatment option.

Conventional medicine has recognized the importance of heredity in causing allergies, and continues to develop better diagnostic tools and more effective medications to both identify the allergen and nullify its effects. But a guaranteed or permanent cure for the sneezing and stuffy and drippy nose of allergic rhinitis is still a long way off.

CHRONIC BRONCHITIS

The primary objective in treating chronic bronchitis is to keep the airways as clear and open as possible. If the person with chronic bronchitis continues to smoke cigarettes, then there is *no* effective treatment program. After smoking has been stopped, a combination of drugs is likely to be prescribed. These may include antibiotics, bronchodilators, and expectorants. The expectorants help to loosen the mucus by decreasing its viscosity. This then increases the efficiency of the cilia on the respiratory mucosa lining the bronchi to remove accumulated secretions. The most frequently used expectorant is guaifenesin, often prescribed as Humibid or Fenesin. Organidin is also an effective expectorant.

Antibiotics are often prescribed for someone with chronic bronchitis during a cold or influenza to prevent a secondary bacterial infection, such as acute bronchitis or pneumonia. These two are similar, but pneumonia is the more severe and serious infection, especially in a patient with underlying chronic bronchitis. The choice of antibiotic will differ from that for a sinusitis patient. Erythromycin, or its newer and stronger derivatives, Zithromax and Biaxin, might be chosen first.

It is not unusual to see acute sinusitis and acute bronchitis occurring together. This condition is called sinobronchitis. The typical symptoms of sinusitis are present along with a persistent (day and night), deep, wet, yellow/green mucusy cough. It is treated in much the same way as a sinus infection; however, Biaxin might be the best choice for an antibiotic.

The basic treatment for chronic bronchitis is similar to that for chronic sinusitis. The objective for the latter condition is to open and drain the obstructed sinus cavity of its thick and/or infected mucus, and for bronchitis you are attempting to do precisely the same thing in the bronchi of the lungs. That's why moisture, especially steam, is also helpful in treating bronchitis. But instead of following the steam with irrigation as I've recommended for sinusitis ("irrigating the lungs" would be the equivalent of drowning), I recommend following it with postural drainage (see pp. 88–90). Postural drainage is one of the best ways to get rid of mucus blocking the airways of your lungs. This procedure enables you to loosen and remove the trapped mucus. I suggest doing it at least once a day. Steaming in the shower, steam room, or with a Steam Inhaler prior to postural drainage will help to thin and loosen the mucus. Drinking plenty of water daily; avoiding the use of cough suppressants; regular use of a humidifier that puts out warm moisture, such as the Bionaire or a steam vaporizer; and avoiding highly polluted, cold, or dry air will also help to thin and remove the mucus. If you must be in an area where there is highly polluted air or strong fumes, wear a special protective mask over your nose and mouth. Some pharmacies and bike shops sell them. There is also a mask called the "Brinks Chemical Respirator" which is effective in filtering fumes and other indoor pollutants. Try to stay away from anything that you know can cause an allergic reaction.

FIGURE 5-3. *Postural Drainage*

Each of the positions shown in the following diagram, either sitting or lying, is designed to allow gravity to assist in draining the mucus from each part of the lungs. Each lung has three parts: an upper, middle, and lower lobe. In each position there is an arrow indicating where an assistant would tap or cup the chest to help jar the mucus loose. This procedure involves cupping the hands as if you were about to clap, then lightly to moderately striking the chest wall, while alternating hands. The rate at which you tap the chest is similar to an average clapping speed. If you are unsure about how to perform this procedure, consult with a respiratory therapist.

UPPER LOBES—A TO F

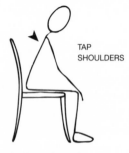

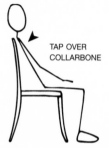

A. Seated in chair. Lean forward about 20°

B. Seated in chair. Lean backward about 20°. You can support lower back with a pillow.

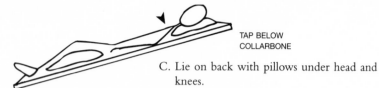

C. Lie on back with pillows under head and knees.

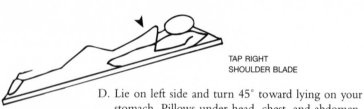

D. Lie on left side and turn 45° toward lying on your stomach. Pillows under head, chest, and abdomen.

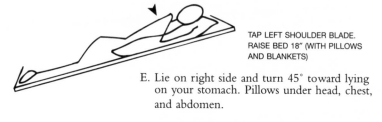

TAP LEFT SHOULDER BLADE. RAISE BED 18″ (WITH PILLOWS AND BLANKETS)

E. Lie on right side and turn 45° toward lying on your stomach. Pillows under head, chest, and abdomen.

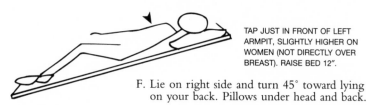

TAP JUST IN FRONT OF LEFT ARMPIT, SLIGHTLY HIGHER ON WOMEN (NOT DIRECTLY OVER BREAST). RAISE BED 12″.

F. Lie on right side and turn 45° toward lying on your back. Pillows under head and back.

MIDDLE LOBE—G

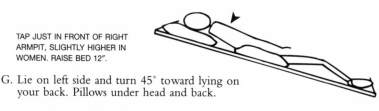

TAP JUST IN FRONT OF RIGHT ARMPIT, SLIGHTLY HIGHER IN WOMEN. RAISE BED 12″.

G. Lie on left side and turn 45° toward lying on your back. Pillows under head and back.

LOWER LOBES—H TO L

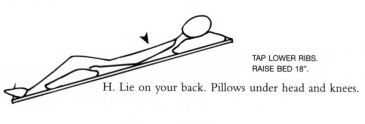

TAP LOWER RIBS. RAISE BED 18″.

H. Lie on your back. Pillows under head and knees.

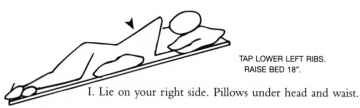

TAP LOWER LEFT RIBS. RAISE BED 18″.

I. Lie on your right side. Pillows under head and waist.

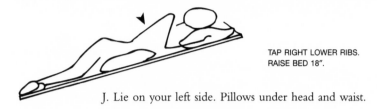

TAP RIGHT LOWER RIBS.
RAISE BED 18″.

J. Lie on your left side. Pillows under head and waist.

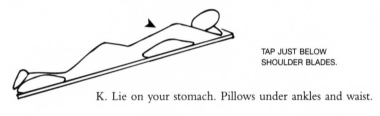

TAP JUST BELOW
SHOULDER BLADES.

K. Lie on your stomach. Pillows under ankles and waist.

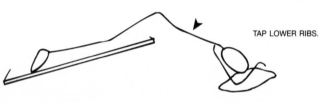

TAP LOWER RIBS.

L. Hang over edge of bed with hips bending 60°.

The conventional medical approach for treating chronic bronchitis can mitigate the symptoms to the extent that the patient adheres to the program. It is a chronic disease and it requires daily persistent treatment. If it is not strictly maintained, as is often the case, the bronchitis slowly progresses. The bronchial walls eventually thicken, and the number of mucous glands increases. The bronchitis sufferer becomes increasingly susceptible to lung infections—acute bronchitis and pneumonia—and the bronchial mucosa becomes more inflamed and secretes a higher volume of thicker mucus. Chronic bronchitis can be incapacitating, often leading to emphysema and eventually, death. Chronic lung disease, consisting primarily of bronchitis and emphysema, is currently the fourth leading cause of death in the United States. Each year it is relentlessly gaining ground on the conditions that hold the top three positions: heart disease, cancer, and stroke.

OTITIS MEDIA
(MIDDLE EAR INFECTION)

The ear is not typically thought of as being a part of the respiratory tract. But the fact that the middle ear space is lined by the same ciliated mucous membrane as the nose and sinuses, and is connected through the eustachian tube (also lined by the same respiratory epithelium) to the back of the nose and throat, technically establishes the middle ear as an integral component of the respiratory tract. It is also impacted by the same factors that adversely affect the nose, sinuses, and lungs, although not as directly.

Middle ear infection, medically known as acute otitis media, is the most common diagnosis in children treated by physicians. Due to the position and anatomy of the eustachian tube, ear infections are very often seen in conjunction with acute sinusitis. The bacteria that most often cause this infection are the same as those responsible for sinus infections. I once heard an ENT physician say that anytime he sees an adult with otitis media, he or she always has an underlying sinus infection.

When otitis media is present, sinusitis might be ignored or even remain unrecognized. These patients are extremely uncomfortable, and their ear pain becomes the focus of attention for both doctor and patient. Young children will usually have a fever above 101°F. The conventional medical treatment of otitis media is usually the same as that of acute sinusitis; therefore, if the diagnosis of sinusitis is missed, the sinus infection will get better anyway. In adults with otitis media, however, I would recommend more regular use of a decongestant than I would for children, and for a longer period of time (three times a day for at least ten days) than I would with sinusitis. This is because adults with middle ear infections routinely complain of "stuffiness" in their ears long after the pain has gone, even after two or three weeks.

Even though the evidence has been mounting that antibiotics

are not effective against most middle ear infections, particularly in children, and may even contribute to recurring infections because they interfere with the body's own immune system, the Centers for Disease Control and Prevention reports that they are prescribed for acute otitis media 99 percent of the time.

In a report released in 1994, the Project on Government Oversight, an independent watchdog group in Washington, said that a researcher at the National Academy of Sciences' Institute of Medicine concluded that antibiotics were no more effective than placebos in treating middle ear infections. Yet the Department of Health and Human Services still recommends antibiotics for ear infections.

Many young children have repeated episodes of acute otitis media, as often as four or five times a year. They usually begin with a cold. After multiple courses of antibiotics, many of these children are referred by their pediatrician or family doctor to an ENT physician, who will very often perform surgery. The procedure is one in which a tube (called a tympanostomy tube) is placed through the eardrum to facilitate drainage from the middle ear space. The number of these surgeries performed every year exceeds even the number of sinus surgeries, and is the most common operation for children that requires general anesthesia.

This is not only unfortunate, in most cases it is also unnecessary. A small but growing number of physicians have recognized that most of the children with recurrent otitis media have a food allergy, usually to milk and dairy products. Other foods that can be responsible for ear infections are eggs, wheat, chocolate, peanuts, corn, and chicken. One ENT specialist in Florida, Dr. Fred Pullen, has claimed that as many as 75 percent of the children referred to him to have tubes inserted in their ears because of chronic ear infections responded so well to eliminating dairy products from their diets that the surgery was unnecessary.

Even *without* considering food allergy as a possible cause of recurrent otitis media, one study has found that about a quarter of middle-ear surgeries to insert tympanostomy tubes in children are "inappropriate." This study, published in the April 1994 issue of the *Journal of the American Medical Association,* also concluded that another one-third of these surgeries may be questionable. This means that several hundred thousand children in the United States may be having tubes surgically inserted in their ears that offer no demonstrated advantage over less-invasive therapies, while also placing them at greater risk for undesirable outcomes.

As you can easily see, there is a clear and consistent pattern with the conventional medical treatment of the most common chronic respiratory diseases. The orientation is entirely on the body and, more specifically, treating the physical symptoms of one particular dysfunctional part. In searching for the causes of disease on only a microscopic, cellular, and tissue level, medical science narrows the focus even further, and usually fails to determine the source of illness. Why does one individual get sick, and another does not? What are the factors that weaken immunity, or maintain health? As a result of the physically limited and narrow disease-oriented scope of medical research, pharmaceutical drugs and surgery have become the primary, and almost only, weapons wielded by physicians in their battle against the enemy—disease. If it's infected or inflamed, then blast it with powerful antibiotics and corticosteroids. If too much histamine is being released, then counterattack with antihistamines. If it's constricted, then open it up with bronchodilators. And if there is an obstruction preventing drainage, then cut it out or create a new opening.

This approach has been extremely successful at saving lives and in effectively treating acute illness. But for the most part, conventional medicine has failed miserably in curing chronic disease. As you've just learned, the overuse of some of these medications has actually contributed to the epidemic of respiratory disease. The narrow perspective of the conventional approach has not allowed for the exploration of alternatives to surgery, resulting in many millions of unnecessary surgical procedures costing billions of dollars. While conventional medicine has brought us miraculous technological advances in treating disease, it has also taken us to the brink of financial ruin. The cost of health care in America in

1995 will exceed $1 trillion. The "business of caring" has become much more of a business, with a lot less caring. Perhaps the time has come to heed the words of former Surgeon General C. Everett Koop, M.D., who continues to warn us: "Beware the medical-pharmaceutical complex!"

Part II

HOLISTIC MEDICINE: THE TREATMENT OF SINUSITIS AND OTHER CHRONIC DIS-EASE

Chapter 6

WHAT IS HOLISTIC MEDICINE?

I f you would rather not learn to live with (or die from) your chronic disease and a diminished quality of life, I would like to take you on a journey into an exciting new frontier of medicine. For the past eight years I have been practicing holistic medicine while treating chronic sinusitis, respiratory disease, and a variety of other so-called "incurable" conditions. The Sinus Survival Program, as outlined in Part II of this book, is the foundation of that practice. *Commitment* to this approach has resulted in a guaranteed significant improvement or cure of the condition being treated. This success stems primarily from the basic *health* orientation of the holistic approach. Rather than focusing on disease and treating its symptoms—they are certainly not ignored, just perceived differently—holistic medicine addresses *causes* while restoring balance and harmony to the whole person. It goes far beyond the "quick fix" or the repair of a "broken part," to an understanding of what can be learned from your physical pain and how to use that knowledge to change your life. My own miserable sinuses have led me to a condition of health I never knew existed. I was guided on this healing path by the words of Hippocrates, "Physician, heal thyself." In the remainder of this book, I'd like to guide you on a similar path leading not only to the healing of your sinuses, lungs, or anything else causing you dis-ease, but to a state of holistic health.

The words "health," "heal," and "holy" all derive from the Anglo-Saxon word *haelen,* meaning "to make whole." Most Americans would probably respond to the question "Are you healthy?" by answering, "I'm not sick, so I must be healthy." Holistic health means more than simply not suffering from any ailment or illness. It is a state of feeling fully alive. It is a condition of wholeness—body, mind, and spirit held in a dynamic state of harmony. It encompasses a balance of environmental, physical, mental, emotional, spiritual, and social health. *The foundation for experiencing this state of well-being is the belief that love is life's most powerful medicine.* More than mere sentiment, love is the very essence of life energy itself. The more alive you feel, the greater your feelings of love for yourself (your body, mind, and spirit) and others. The greater love's degree of unconditionality, the more powerful its healing potential.

Holistic health is also the end result of the practice of holistic medicine. The American Holistic Medical Association (AHMA) defines holistic medicine as "a philosophy of medical care which emphasizes personal responsibility and fosters a cooperative doctor-patient relationship. It encompasses all safe modalities of diagnosis and treatment while emphasizing the whole person—physical, mental, emotional and spiritual." Holistic medicine is not limited to any particular medical specialty or type of treatment. It incorporates elements of many types of medicine, including allopathic (whose practitioners are M.D.s), osteopathic (D.O.s), naturopathic (N.D.s), chiropractic (D.C.s), Chinese (O.M.D.s), environmental, and preventive. The active members of the AHMA are all M.D.s and D.O.s representing almost every medical specialty, but the majority are primary care physicians—family physicians, internists, and pediatricians. Associate members of the AHMA must be registered or certified in the state in which they practice. Among these holistic practitioners are naturopathic physicians, chiropractors, doctors of Chinese medicine, homeopaths, nurses, dentists, podiatrists, psychologists, social workers, physical therapists, dieticians, pharmacists, optometrists, physician assistants, respiratory therapists, speech therapists, and veterinarians. All members adhere to the principles of holistic medical practice (see Table 6-1). A physician practicing "alternative medicine" is not necessarily considered a holistic physician merely because he or she is treating patients with a therapy beyond the scope of conventional medicine, such as nutrition, homeopathy, or acupuncture. Unless the practitioner alone, or as part of a therapeutic team, is treating the whole person—body, mind, and spirit—he or she is *not* practicing holistic medicine.

The holistic practitioner and patient share responsibility by working together to facilitate the healing process. The word "doctor" derives from a Latin word meaning "teacher." Rather than merely being a fixer of the broken part of the body, a holistic doctor becomes a teacher of health, enabling patients to repair themselves and to take better care of their environment, body, mind, emotions, spirit, and relationships. Hippocrates' command to physicians to heal themselves was an invitation to the aspiring healer to discover the power of the healing process in the only way it can be discovered: through personal experience. He was also saying that if physicians are to become effective health educators, the best way to teach is to practice what you preach.

Table 6-1

Principles of Holistic Medical Practice

Adopted by the American Holistic Medical Association March 9, 1993

1. Holistic physicians embrace a variety of safe, effective options in diagnosis and treatment, including
   1) education for lifestyle changes and self-care;
   2) complementary approaches; and
   3) conventional drugs and surgery.
2. Searching for the underlying causes of disease is preferable to treating symptoms alone.

3. Holistic physicians expend as much effort in establishing what kind of patient has a disease as they do in establishing what kind of disease a patient has.

4. It is preferable to diagnose and treat patients as unique individuals rather than as members of a disease category.

5. When possible, lifestyle modifications are preferable to drugs and surgery as initial therapeutic options.

6. Prevention is preferable to treatment and is usually *more* cost-effective. The *most* cost-effective approach evokes the patient's own innate healing capabilities.

7. Illness is viewed as a manifestation of a dysfunction of the whole person, not as an isolated event.

8. In most situations encouragement of patient autonomy is preferable to decisions imposed by physicians.

9. The ideal physician-patient relationship considers the needs, desires, awareness, and insight of the patient as well as those of the physician.

10. The quality of the relationship established between physician and patient is a major determinant of healing outcomes.

11. Physicians significantly influence patients by their example.

12. Illness, pain, and the dying process can be learning opportunities for patients and physicians.

13. Holistic physicians encourage patients to evoke the healing power of love, hope, humor, and enthusiasm and to release the toxic consequences of hostility, shame, greed, depression, and prolonged fear, anger, and grief.

14. Unconditional love is life's most powerful medicine. Physicians strive to adopt an attitude of unconditional love for patients, themselves, and other practitioners.

15. Holistic or optimal health is much more than the absence of sickness. It is the conscious pursuit of the highest qualities of the spiritual, mental, emotional, physical, environmental, and social aspects of the human experience.

In addressing causes, the holistic approach does not often lend itself to the "quick fix" to which our society has become so accustomed. Whether our need is for food, energy, information, entertainment, transportation, communication, or health care, we look to satisfy it in the fastest, simplest, and most effortless way. Science and technology have attempted to keep pace with our desire for speed and ease, and indeed, they have performed incredible, at times almost miraculous, feats that have allowed an ease of living never before experienced in human history. However, there is a price to be paid for all of this comfort. Technology is helping us to destroy our environment—to pollute our air, poison our food and water, deplete our soil, thin our protective ozone layer, decimate our forests at the rate of one acre every second, and cause the extinction of nearly 100 species of plants and animals *daily*! Our own species, *Homo sapiens,* might not be far behind.

Sinus disease might be the proverbial canary in the coal mine. (Miners often take canaries with them into mines to use as an early-warning sign of oxygen depletion or of the presence of toxic gases. If the canaries die, the miner knows it is time to get out of the mine.) There is already overwhelming evidence that the health of the entire human respiratory tract is rapidly deteriorating. More than one-third of all Americans suffer from some form of respiratory disease, and more people are dying from asthma, chronic bronchitis, emphysema, and lung cancer than ever before. By destroying the quality of our air and our environment, we appear to be in the process of destroying ourselves. Many of us are becoming "human canaries," and it is time to get out of the "coal mine" and change the way we live as individuals and as a society.

CAUSES

Holistic medicine emphasizes harmony and integration within individuals, between them and their community, and with the planet itself. To address the burgeoning state of disharmony and imbalance that exists today both within our bodies and on the earth, we must begin by confronting the causes of our dis-ease and restoring our own health. I strongly believe that *air pollution* is the primary cause of the epidemic of respiratory disease. The mucous membrane lining the entire respiratory tract from the nose to the lungs is subjected to a relentless assault of toxic pollutants with almost every one of our 23,000 daily breaths.

If we were able to maintain a strong immune system, we might be able to withstand the onslaught of the pollutants without getting infected, allergic, asthmatic, or bronchitic. However, *the combination of environmental and emotional toxins has significantly weakened the human immune system.* In recent years we have developed a number of disorders related to an impaired immune system. These diseases, which were unknown or quite rare as recently as fifteen years ago, are now turning into epidemics. The Epstein-Barr virus, the cause of mononucleosis, is now responsible for chronic fatigue syndrome. Besides the four respiratory diseases (asthma, chronic bronchitis, emphysema, and lung cancer), herpes simplex infections, candidiasis (the subject of Chapter 9), "ecologic illness," lupus (systemic lupus erythematosus), multiple sclerosis, and AIDS (acquired immunodeficiency syndrome) are all examples of this phenomenon. As you will soon learn in the section about psychoneuroimmunology, emotional stress can also have a profound impact on immune function. This is not a new development, but it is a relatively recent scientific discovery. The heightened stress levels pervading the planet, together with the environmental pollution, seem to have created a potentially devastating situation for normal immune function.

As more people contract these illnesses, the job of the primary care physician is becoming even more challenging than it already was. Managed care (HMOs, PPOs) is rapidly becoming the dominant force in America's health care system. The foundation of these medical insurance companies is built upon primary care physicians and the concepts of cost-effective and preventive medicine. Although they profess to want better health for their subscribers (HMO = Health Maintenance Organization), like any other business, their chief objective is to make money. One of the essential ways of attaining that goal is by insisting that all patients be seen first by a primary care physician. These family doctors, internists, and pediatricians are often overwhelmed with too many patients and can be financially penalized if they refer too many people to specialists. They have neither the time nor, in most cases, the training to teach their patients how to maintain good health. (Medical school is almost entirely focused on the diagnosis and treatment of disease.) The result is that many physicians attempt to reduce medical costs by prescribing medication over the phone, thereby avoiding an office visit. They also save money for the insurance company by minimizing referrals to specialists and caring for more seriously ill patients than they did previously. The result of both of these common practices is that *antibiotics, corticosteroids, and beta-agonists are often over-prescribed,* which can lead to antibiotic-resistant supergerms, candidiasis, immune suppression, and uncontrolled asthma. This disturbing development is, sadly, another major contributor to the epidemic of respiratory disease, and has also resulted in significantly diminishing the quality of health care in this country.

MIND-BODY MEDICINE

Conventional medicine has been extremely effective in treating acute illness—bacterial infections, allergy and asthma attacks, accidents, and life-threatening medical and surgical emergencies. But it is the prohibitive cost of treating chronic disease that has been most responsible for the financial crisis in health care today. The word "chronic" has become a medical euphemism for "incurable," while patients suffering with these conditions fill the offices of primary care physicians for symptom treatment. In the majority of these cases, successful medical treatment simply means that symptoms are (1) alleviated until the body's natural healing mechanism and immune system can finish the job, as with colds, sore throats, and most viral infections; (2) relieved and controlled with long-term medication, surgery, diet, and other measures, as in chronic sinusitis, arthritis, diabetes, high blood pressure, and allergies; or (3) variably relieved with drugs and surgery, as in many forms of cancer; Parkinson's, Alzheimer's, and other neurologic diseases; and AIDS.

As medicine begins its shift from a disease- to a health-oriented approach, the opportunities for curing chronic disease have increased tremendously. Herbert Benson, M.D., director of the Mind/Body Clinic in the Department of Behavioral Medicine at the Harvard University School of Medicine, has shown how relaxation techniques can treat high blood pressure, migraine headaches, and many other common and chronic ailments. He has also documented the healing power of prayer, which I address again in Chapter 12. Bernie Siegel, M.D., of the Yale University School of Medicine, a past president of the AHMA and the author of the best-seller *Love, Medicine and Miracles,* has had extraordinary results in treating his cancer patients with holistic medicine. C. Norman Shealy, M.D., a neurosurgeon, cofounder and original president of the AHMA, and co-author of *The Creation of Health,* has seen remarkable results for more than eighteen years in the holistic treatment of chronic pain. Using a holistic approach, Dean Ornish, M.D., at the University of California School of Medicine at San Francisco, has been able to *reverse* coronary artery disease (the leading cause of death in the United States) in his patients—something that has never before been demonstrated. He describes this method in his book *Dr. Dean Ornish's Program for Reversing Heart Disease.*

If holistic medicine has been shown as effective in treating migraine headaches, high blood pressure, chronic pain, cancer, and heart disease, surely it also can be used to treat the nation's most common chronic disease: chronic sinusitis, as well as asthma, allergies, and chronic bronchitis. In fact, all of these conditions respond quite well to holistic treatment. The following pages give a brief description of my approach to holistic health and the holistic medical treatment of chronic sinusitis and the three other respiratory conditions. Each component of health warrants an entire book, and, indeed, makes reference to several relevant works. The program I present here is one I have taught for the past eight years in the treatment of sinus disease and other chronic conditions. Its focus is on learning to experience greater health and well-being in body, mind, emotions, spirit, and relationships. As by-products of this course of study and of treating the whole person, not only do sinuses, nose, and lungs feel better, but patients feel a greater sense of vitality and enjoyment of life than they have experienced before.

Learning to become your own healer requires a commitment to loving yourself, a willingness to change, an open mind, time, effort, and patience. You can choose to do as much or as little as feels comfortable to you. Many of my patients have experienced great relief from their sinus symptoms after working on just the physical component. However, if you are interested in curing a chronic disease, you must go further. Trust your intuition and remember that, as the "physician" directing this program, you are following an inexact prescription; therefore, you can't make mistakes.

Following the chapter on environment, physical fitness is the first of five aspects of holistic health that will be discussed. None of the others seems to be as easy or quick to change as the physical (and believe me, I've tried). Yet the cure for chronic sinusitis and any other chronic disease lies in healing not only the physical but the less tangible parts of ourselves: the mind, emotions, spirit, and relationships. All of these aspects of health lie beyond the scope of our five senses.

The nonphysical aspect of my practice is based on *psychoneuroimmunology,* the complicated interplay between the body and the mind, which derives its name from *psycho,* the brain, *neuro,* the nervous system, and *immunology,* the study of the immune system. This is the scientific basis of holistic medicine. It has also been called mind-body medicine or behavioral medicine. Research has confirmed that our thoughts, beliefs, attitudes, emotions, and relationships (both with other people and with a higher power) can either strengthen or weaken our immune system. This process occurs in the transmission of messenger molecules (neuropeptides) through the nervous system to be received by the immune system. Many scientists believe this feedback mechanism is so sensitive that they are now referring to the immune system as "a circulating nervous system." In the practice of mind-body medicine, the mind aspect encompasses mental, emotional, spiritual, and social health. The condition referred to as stress or emotional stress can result from an imbalance in any or all of these four aspects of health. A critical factor in the cause of chronic sinusitis and all other dis-ease is this hidden, largely unconscious part of ourselves.

As I practice medicine, I see myself as a teacher. The course of study I teach is holistic health. Many of my "students" (patients) come to "class" monthly for an extended consultation. Initially they come for the treatment of a chronic disease or with the desire to experience a greater degree of health. The majority of these students are chronic sinus sufferers.

My "curriculum" has evolved over the past eight years. It was designed to implement the principles of mind-body medicine and to help others practice holistic medicine on themselves, as I am doing on myself. There is no doubt that each of us has the potential to become our own best healer. In order to assume greater responsibility for our own health, however, we first need to educate ourselves.

What follows is a set of healthy options from which to choose. Using your intuition to refine and personalize this process of self-healing, you will experience a greater degree of physical fitness, vigor and vitality, peace of mind, ability to use your gifts, joy and exhilaration, awareness of and ability to express feelings, intimacy with others, a greater connection to God and nature, and very healthy sinuses and lungs. *You will become more aware of what feels good and what doesn't, and you will learn to make choices that are life enhancing. You are, in essence, learning to love yourself in body, mind, and spirit, and in so doing will be better able to give and receive love.* This program is based on the belief that love is our most powerful healer. Each of us is the best person to administer that medicine to ourselves. It is an inexpensive drug without unpleasant side effects, and one on which you cannot overdose.

In the chapters that follow, you will be provided with a prescription for improving six components of human health, while treating each of the primary causes of the four chronic respiratory diseases. I have referred to several books for those who would like to explore these areas in greater depth. I have tried to simplify each component and have suggested "exercises" to help you find your own path to a greater level of physical, mental, emotional, spiritual, and social fitness. These exercises must be practiced regularly in order to be effective. (However, if a particular exercise feels too uncomfortable to you, don't do it.) If you are willing to wait and practice—remember, it took years for you to develop your current state of health—I promise you not only that they will all work, but that every one of them will feel good. Keep in mind that although this is a course with a lot of homework, there are no exams or grades, so enjoy yourself!

You will first learn how to heal the sensitive and "wounded" mucous membranes, by nurturing them with optimal air and moisture and removing irritants from your environment. There are numerous methods to strengthen a weakened immune system and many treatment options in lieu of antibiotics and other powerful drugs with potentially harmful side effects. Although I infrequently prescribe most of these medications or recommend surgery, there are instances in which they are the preferable choice. *Holistic medicine is not an alternative to conventional medicine, but a complement.* It is also the most therapeutically sound and cost-effective approach to the treatment of chronic disease that I've found in twenty-five years of practicing medicine. By taking responsibility for your own health, you become not only your own healer, but a highly skilled practitioner of preventive medicine as well. Before the turn of the century, as holistic medicine becomes conventional medicine's newest specialty, the model for self-care presented on the following pages will become an integral part of America's evolving health care system.

Chapter 7

HOW TO HELP YOUR SINUSES BY CHANGING YOUR ENVIRONMENT

Over the past six years I have met with air filtration, humidification, negative ionization, and indoor air pollution experts; allergists; specialists in environmental medicine; and ecological architects. With their guidance and their state-of-the-art technology, I have learned a great deal about environmental health. The information in this chapter is a result of that education.

Environmental health is a condition of respect and appreciation for your home, community, nature, and the earth. It is a relationship of harmony with your environment—neither harming nor being harmed by, while enhancing and being enlivened by your surroundings.

There is nothing more important to human health and survival than the air we breathe. The sinuses and the nose, our first line of defense against unhealthy air, are a sensitive gauge of air quality. Ideal quality is rated by clarity (freedom from pollutants), humidity (between 35 and 45 percent), temperature (between 65° and 85°F), oxygen content (21 percent of total volume and 100 percent saturation), and negative ion content (3,000 to 6,000 .001-micron ions per cubic centimeter). Air that is clean, moist, warm, oxygen rich, and high in negative ions is the healthiest air a human being can breathe.

Not only are we dependent on oxygen for survival, but every part of the human body thrives with a maximum supply of oxygen. If your respiratory tract is defective because of a nasal, sinus, or lung ailment, or if the amount of oxygen available in the air is relatively low (for example, air high in carbon monoxide, air at higher altitudes, or stale indoor air), your body is receiving less than its optimal requirement of oxygen.

Negative ions are air molecules that have excess electrons. Negative ions vitalize or freshen the air we breathe. The earth itself is a natural negative-ion generator. Health spas have always been located in areas high in negative ions (3,000 to 20,000 per cubic centimeter of air), such as along seacoasts, near rushing streams and waterfalls, in mountainous areas, and in pine forests (pine needles cause negative ions to be generated in the surrounding air). Studies have shown that negative ions increase the sweeping motion of the cilia on the respiratory mucosa, and subsequently enhance the movement of mucus and the clearing or filtering of inhaled pollutants. They also help to reduce pain, heal burns, suppress mold and bacterial growth, and stimulate plant growth, and they contribute greatly to our sense of well-being and comfort.

Positive ions, on the other hand, are air molecules lacking electrons. Pollen can carry fifty or more positive charges per grain of pollen. This positive charge slows the cilia and the clearing of mucus, and in so doing can cause some degree of nasal congestion. Most man-made pollutants result from combustion processes (auto/truck exhaust, smokestacks, cigarette smoke, etc.), which leave the pollutants with a positive charge. Heating and ventilation systems tend to produce air containing an excess of positive ions. Aircraft cabins have been tested and found to contain an excessively high amount of positive ions. This obviously contributes to the "stuffy" feeling of airplane air, and also helps to explain why so many of my patients have developed sinus infections following air travel.

The negative ion content of indoor air can be as low as 10 to 200 negative ions per cubic centimeter. This is considered to be "ion depleted" air and is a significant component of "sick building syndrome." Ion depleted air is also created by heating/cooling systems; window air conditioners; air cleaners (including HEPA filters), which "scrub" negative ions from the air; and the screens of television sets and computers, which have a high positive charge that draws negative ions out of the air and neutralizes them. Most of the factors in our environment responsible for depleting the beneficial negative ions also produce an excess of unhealthy positive ions.

The majority of Americans spend 90 percent of their time indoors, where, the EPA says, the air can be as much as 100 times more polluted than outdoor air. Few of us live in clean, moist environments that are warm year-round; even fewer live in the mountains, on a beach, or in the woods. For the 92 million people whose sinuses, nose, and lungs are already feeling the pain that comes from breathing unhealthy air, and for anyone else who wants to enjoy optimum health, here are some ways to minimize the risks of breathing poor-quality air and to prevent respiratory disease.

LOCATION

Where we live, work, play, or otherwise spend our time is critical to our health. If you are considering a move and need help in evaluating a potential location, use this list from Richard L. Crowther's book *Indoor Air: Risks and Remedies:*

- Locate in houses and buildings that minimize the impact of outdoor air pollution.
- Locate in a city, town, or county that has minimal air pollution.
- Locate on a hill rather than in a valley, where pollution is more apt to concentrate.
- Do not locate near a major highway or traffic intersection.
- Do not locate next to a parking lot.
- Do not locate downwind from a power plant, chemical plant, or processing plant.
- Do not locate near industrial operations.
- Do not locate near businesses that emit pollutants.

- Do not locate near a railroad line that carries hazardous materials.
- Do not locate near airfields.
- Do not locate on land farmed with pesticides and chemical fertilizers.
- Locate away from agricultural fields that are sprayed.
- Do not live under or near high-voltage power lines.
- Locate away from stagnant waterways.
- Locate out of the air pollution or "seepage" range of oil or gas wells.
- Locate a safe distance from any mining operations.
- Locate close to a park, near a forest, or within a natural setting.
- Locate in a small, healthful rural or seacoast community.
- Consider the effect of altitude on air quality.
- Consider prevailing daily and seasonal wind patterns.
- Before moving to a city, review an air quality record of the past several years.
- In urban or rural locations, consider sites for passive solar orientation and exposure.
- South-sloping sites are preferable for drainage and solar advantage.
- Avoid being in a "shadow path" during winter months in a cold climate.
- Avoid sites with high levels of radon or radioactivity.
- Before buying a property, get soils, radon, and water tests (if a well is planned).
- Check municipal water quality.

In addition, if allergies are a problem for you, it would be helpful to check with the local allergy society on the predominant allergens in that area. I would also suggest living there for at least one month before making the commitment to move.

It is unlikely that all of these locational criteria can be met, but they can provide a basis for a thorough evaluation. If you are going to relocate and have the freedom to choose, avoid the following regions: Southern California, the Northeast, and the

Texas Gulf Coast. The healthiest air can be found along the West Coast (with the distinct exception of the Los Angeles metropolitan area and southward), rural areas along the Gulf coast (other than Texas), and the west coast of Florida. I used to think that Hawaii was the optimum healthy environment until I heard from a *Sinus Survival* reader living on the big island of Hawaii. He told me that both he and his wife have recently developed terrible sinus problems, as have many of their friends. For nearly ten years the active volcanoes on that island have been spewing lava (600,000 cubic yards per day) and volcanic ash. When the lava hits the ocean water, it produces hydrochloric acid. This in combination with the ash has created a serious problem of toxic visible pollution that is threatening to ruin "paradise," or at least the respiratory tracts of many of its residents, and some of the aesthetic value of Hawaii as well. Apparently this volcanic pollution is, to some degree, affecting most of the Hawaiian islands and has resulted in many people moving back to the mainland.

ECOLOGICAL ARCHITECTURE

If you are contemplating the construction of a new home, the concept of ecological architecture could help considerably in creating a healthy environment. *Ecology* is defined in Webster's *New World Dictionary* as "the branch of biology that deals with the relationship between living organisms and their environment." Used as a modifier for the word *architecture,* it simply means the design of a dwelling that is sensitive to human health and gentle to the earth. Once we have considered the microclimate and the site, our biologic needs, behavior patterns, and, most important, our budgetary limitations, nature will then dictate the design. Self-sufficiency through use of sun, air, earth, and water for heating, cooling, ventilation, and even electrical power is a realistic goal of an ecological design.

Common objectives regarding construction methods and materials include

- avoiding the use of plastic or other materials made of toxic ingredients that harmfully outgas (give off toxins and/or fumes) in the indoor environment;
- the use of nontoxic natural materials in preference to synthetic materials;
- design concern for sensitivities, allergies, or chronic health problems;
- concern that nature's ecologic sustainability and well-being should not be diminished by what is built; and
- a responsibility to conceive, design, build, and furnish a home or building to a "healthy home" ecological ethic.

This is a holistic approach emphasizing the ecological bond between site and architecture. Preservation and wise use of our planet's resources in construction and throughout the lifetime of a home is fundamental to ecological design. For the sinus sufferer, a home must be clean, moist, warm, and oxygen and negative ion rich. The fact that it is designed in harmony with the atmosphere and the earth makes this an environmentally healthy concept.

I fully appreciate that most readers of this book will neither move nor design their own home as a result of what they read here. However, I want to present as many environmental treatment options as possible. Each can have a profound impact on your state of health and ultimately your quality of life.

HEALTHY HOMES

You can create an oasis of healthy indoor air in your own home. In the desert an oasis provides water. In the sea of hazardous air in which we live, a healthy home or business can provide an oasis in which to breathe life-enhancing air.

Solving the problem of indoor air pollution entails both treatment and prevention. There is a company in Denver, called Healthy Habitats, that has been on the leading edge of this field for more than seven years. The owner of the company, Carl

Grimes, has worked with me and a number of my patients to transform our unhealthy homes and offices into healthy ones. The procedures and techniques he employs adhere to the following guidelines:

1. Prevention—avoid bringing pollutants into the home and workplace.
2. Identify the source and develop a plan for isolating or removing the pollutant from the "breathing zone," or the surrounding area from which you obtain your breathing air; e.g., an infant's breathing zone includes the floor and carpeting.
3. Reduce ambient pollution with ventilation, filtration, and ionization.

Grimes considers the three primary sources of pollution to be:

1. Particulates—dust, pollen, dander, construction debris, and smoke.
2. Microorganisms—bacteria, viruses, molds, and dust mites.
3. Chemicals—(refer to Table 2-1, pages 21–22), personal care products, cleaning products, office equipment, and building/construction materials.

The type of treatment depends upon the type of pollution. For example, HEPA filtration might be used for particulates, charcoal for chemicals, and the drying of a wet crawl space could be the best option for eliminating microbes. Ozone has also been effective for persistent microorganisms.

Several excellent books are available on the subject of healthy homes. Those that I am familiar with are: *The Nontoxic Home and Office,* by Debra Lynn Dadd (Jeremy P. Tarcher, Inc.); *The Healthy House,* by John Bower (Lyle Stuart Inc.); *Your Home, Your Health and Well-Being,* by David Rousseau (Ten Speed Press); *Chemical Exposures: Low Levels and High Stakes,* by Claudia Miller and Nicholas Ashford (Van Nostrand Reinhold).

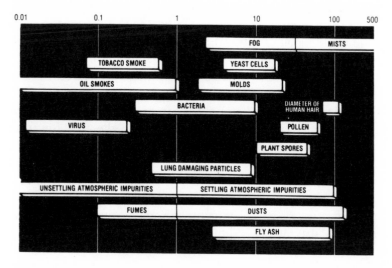

FIGURE 7-1. *Relative Size of Common Air Contaminants*

AIR CLEANERS AND NEGATIVE-ION GENERATORS

As many as one million hospital admissions a year are attributed to poor indoor air quality. In recent years, as the EPA and private health organizations have publicized the problem of indoor air pollution, we have seen a proliferation of several hundred types of air cleaners, almost as many as there are indoor air pollutants. According to Michael Berry, Ph.D., former manager of the EPA's Indoor Air Project, the most potentially harmful pollutants are radon and the "biologicals," including pollen, mold, plant spores, dust mites, bacteria, and viruses. The pollutants most harmful to the respiratory tract are less than one micron in size. Regardless of their origin, size, or health-damaging effects, air pollutants can be described as free-floating particles in the air. Figure 7-1 shows the specific size ranges of the most common pollutants. The unit of measurement used for tiny air particles is the micron. An average hair strand is 100 microns thick, and about 400 1-micron particles would fit into the dot over the "i" in the word *micron*. The primary job of air cleaners is to remove as many of these particles as possible, the biologicals as well as the combustion products, particulates, chemicals, fumes, and odors (see Table 2-1, pp. 21–22). Radon, if present, requires the sealing of basement cracks and improvement of basement ventilation. Most air cleaners do not remove radon from the air. However, some air cleaners with high particle removal efficiency (HEPA, etc.) can remove some of the radon "daughters" (attached radon) that are in particulate form. A study at the Harvard School of Public Health determined that a negative-ion generator is a highly effective means of removing the attached fraction of radon (the radon daughters), although it does not reduce the unattached (gaseous) fraction of radon.

The strategy for solving the problem of indoor air pollution involves air cleaning and improved ventilation. Air cleaning devices can include furnace filters, portable stand-alone units, and negative ion generators. The efficiency of air cleaners is evaluated by their ability to filter a certain percentage of a certain size of pollutant. The HEPA filter (an acronym for high efficiency particulate arrestor) removes 97 percent of all 0.3 micron particulates and larger. This includes pollen, plant spores, most animal dander, dust, wood, and tobacco smoke, fumes, bacteria, and some viruses. This type of filter is standard equipment for most hospital operating suites, and is found in many of the more expensive free-standing air cleaners. It requires a strong fan or a booster fan to move air through it due to its increased efficiency.

Negative-ion generators were originally designed to restore a more natural and beneficial level of negative ions to indoor air. In the course of their use for biological benefit, it was discovered that free-floating ions quickly attach to airborne particles and cause them to agglomerate and precipitate from the air, or be drawn to grounded surfaces such as walls, metal surfaces, etc. Ionizers are highly effective air cleaners, removing particles as small as .001 micron, which would include viruses, dust, pollen, cigarette smoke, and all other airborne particulate pollutants.

Compared to air cleaners with fans or blowers, ionizers are more likely to be operated full-time since they are totally silent (no fan), and consume only pennies of electricity per month.

However, in order to increase the speed with which an ionizer cleans the air, many manufacturers produce ionizers with excessive ion output. This has two undesirable effects: (1) The ion density established by these ionizers exceeds many times the natural range found outdoors, resulting in much the same adverse effects as breathing air with too few negative ions. A well-designed negative-ion generator will generate enough ions to be effective but will not exceed an upper limit that would make it biologically undesirable. (2) An excessively high ion density also causes a significant amount of pollutants to be driven to the walls and other grounded surfaces, resulting in the buildup of a dirty residue. Again, a well-designed ion generator will minimize such "plating," and this effect can be further reduced by placing the ionizer at least two feet from the nearest wall.

It has been my good fortune, and that of my patients, to have worked with a "pioneer" in negative-ion technology. For nearly twenty-five years, Rex Coppom, owner of Air Tech International in Boulder, Colorado, has been developing state-of-the-art negative-ion generators. For almost four years many of my patients have been using his Sinus Survival Air Vitalizer, a small unit that will clean the air of a 150-square-foot room and maintain an ideal level of negative ions. It costs $150, which is about one-half to one-third the price of a HEPA room air cleaner that is comparable in its cleaning efficiency but has no negative ions. I have received many testimonials about its beneficial effects—dramatic headache relief, diminished nasal congestion, cessation of snoring, better sleep, more energy, fewer allergy and asthma attacks, and diminished odor and symptoms resulting from secondhand cigarette smoke. I was amazed at how quickly it cleared the smoke from my kitchen during an oven-cleaning session that went somewhat awry. Rex is currently in the process of developing ionization equipment for automobiles and aircraft cabins.

Electronic air cleaners (both central and free-standing) produce positive ions as they filter the air. On their first day of operation they are 85 percent efficient on all 1-micron particles and larger, but in order to maintain that efficiency they require cleaning every two weeks. For most of us, this makes them impractical and inconvenient. They also produce ozone, which, as discussed in Chapter 2, can be a potential health hazard.

To obtain a furnace filter, go to a hardware or building-supply store. Many of them carry the 3M pleated filter, under the brand names Filtret and Electret. These are excellent furnace filters and cost about $15. They should be replaced every one to two months during the winter and while central air-conditioners are being run regularly. They are far more efficient than the $2 to $4 varieties found in supermarkets. Columbus Industries will also be offering an effective and inexpensive (both $8 and $14) furnace filter by October 1995. Similar to the 3M filter and slightly more efficient, it is called "The Magnet," and will be available at Sears stores.

The Dupont Wizard dustcloth is an interesting new product that does a better job of dusting than can be obtained from liquid or spray dust cleaners. They are used dry, can be washed, and cost $2.

AIR DUCT CLEANING

When the air duct system of my thirteen-year-old home was cleaned for the first time, I was amazed at what emanated from the ducts after two hours of high-intensity vacuuming. I thought to myself, "It's no wonder I suffered with sinus problems for so long!" If the air ducts are filthy, it is nearly impossible for your furnace filter to clean the air in your home. After the air is filtered, it still has to travel through the ducts before you breathe it. I recommend air duct cleaning as part of the environmental treatment program. Depending on the size of your home, an air duct cleaning service, using good equipment, could cost between $200 and $250. To find this type of company in your city, look in the Yellow Pages under "Furnaces, Cleaning and Repairing."

CARPET CLEANING

Carpets are one of the most common sources of indoor air pollutants. They are excellent traps and hold onto dust, pollen, and microorganisms. While this helps to keep those particles out of the breathing zone, their gradual accumulation can become great enough to create a sustainable culture of bacteria, yeast, dust mites, and mold. In fact, many allergists recommend that their patients dispose of all their carpets.

While it is true that carpets harbor pollutants, it is possible to keep them clean. This poses a challenge to the homemaker. Conventional vacuum cleaners are designed to remove and retain the visible dirt, which means particles greater than 10 microns. Most of the particles and microorganisms that are too small to be seen are also smaller than the pores in the vacuum cleaner bag. This allows most of them to blow through the bag and into the room, settling back onto the carpets and furniture. If a forced-air heating system is running, the airborne particles can be drawn into the air ducts, contributing to their contamination as well. Also, as the bag fills, airflow decreases, causing uneven cleaning.

To prevent these problems I suggest a vacuum cleaner that uses either a HEPA-type filter or water-capture. Either one removes even sub-visible dust and bacteria from the air. The water-capture types also have a continuously maximum airflow because they won't clog like a bag or filter. Both of these vacuums are expensive, costing in the vicinity of $500 to $1,000.

I've recently learned about a much less expensive alternative. Dupont Hysurf vacuum cleaner bags have 1-micron pores, and cost only $5. They appear to have the equivalent cleaning efficiency of the $500-plus "allergy" vacuum cleaners. Their major problem is that they are difficult to find. Some janitorial supply houses and medical supply stores have them. They can also be obtained from Healthy Habitats.

Many people have their carpets professionally cleaned. However, due to their chemical composition, the most common cleaning agents are often worse than having dirty carpets. Alcohols, petroleum distillates, ammonia, dry-cleaning substances, and scents often cause headaches, mental "fuzziness," lethargy, and a general feeling of discomfort. Cleaning-agent residues may often cause respiratory irritation.

Before contracting with a carpet cleaner, check his references and insist on a non-scented cleaning agent that uses no petroleum distillates, alcohol, ammonia, dry-cleaning-type chemicals or enzymes, and has no suds that can be left in the carpet. Check his work to be sure he leaves no damp areas. This ensures maximum removal of all agents and enhances drying time. If the carpet stays wet for several days, bacteria and molds can grow rapidly.

VENTILATION, OXYGEN, AND PLANTS

All indoor spaces, whether residential, commercial, industrial, or recreational, require some type of ventilation to provide breathable air for occupants, to furnish combustion air for cooking and heating, and to remove stale air filled with toxins and particulates. Commercial buildings are required by code to have even more efficient ventilation systems than residences. The American Society of Heating, Refrigerating and Air-Conditioning Engineers (ASHRAE) says that air should be replaced at the rate of 15 cubic feet per minute per person, but most systems fall below this minimum standard.

Improving ventilation will help relieve indoor air pollution as long as the outdoor air isn't dirtier than the air it is replacing. Local pollution sources, such as fumes from toxic waste leakage, wood burning, a neighboring industrial plant, a heavily trafficked highway, or crop spraying can render outdoor air unacceptable for indoor ventilation. Several days a year, Los Angeles residents are advised to keep all windows and doors closed and ventilation ducts shut to prevent the heavily polluted outdoor air from entering homes and businesses. In areas like this, it becomes a challenge to balance the health benefit of highly oxygenated outdoor air and the liability of the pollutants that come with it. Outdoor aerobic exercise presents a similar dilemma. If you live in a heavily polluted environment, I recommend exercising outside and ventilating your home and office well when outdoor air is good, but exercise indoors and keep windows and doors closed during periods of heavy pollution.

Air-conditioning systems are a helpful means of ventilation for people with respiratory and allergy problems. These systems remove excess moisture from the air, lowering its temperature. In less humid conditions there is a reduction of molds and spores, and with the windows closed there is also a marked decrease in pollen from the outdoors. Air conditioning, however, does deplete negative ions from the air.

Natural cross-ventilation is effective in reducing indoor air pollution if the placement of the intake vents is low and the outlets for the flow-through air are high. Operable windows on commercial buildings and a good location for the outdoor air intake—away from garage entrances or loading docks—are also important factors in improving indoor air quality. Mechanical ventilation with exhaust fans can certainly help in removing indoor pollutants, but such fans are most efficient when used in a confined space. Private offices or single-occupant rooms where smoking, cooking, and other fume-producing activities take place are ideal environments for mechanical ventilation.

Rooms producing commercial toxic or odoriferous fumes; spaces subject to bacterial and viral contamination, such as rest rooms; and indoor areas that present specific respiratory hazards all need optimized ventilation. Mold is a special problem in moist conditions. Adequate ventilation along with sunshine can help to reduce moisture and subsequently suppress mold.

The technology of ventilation can be complex, but the basic principle of displacing interior air with outdoor air and increasing the rate of fresh air flow is critical to treating the problem of indoor air pollution. Besides natural cross-ventilation and exhaust fans, other devices used to enhance ventilation and indoor air quality are air-to-air heat exchangers, makeup air units, attic fans, vortex fans, and ceiling fans. Remember that even if the "fresh" air is filthy, an effective air cleaner combined with good ventilation is still a winning combination.

Adequate ventilation not only helps reduce indoor air pollution, but is the primary source of indoor oxygen. Plants can offer an aesthetically pleasant secondary source. Although the oxygen output from indoor plants is not great, plants with large leaf surfaces that grow rapidly are capable of enhancing air quality. Attached greenhouses and atria filled with plants that effectively absorb carbon dioxide and oxygenate the air (spider plants do this very well) can improve the indoor environment while humidifying the air.

In recent years, studies conducted at the John Stennis Space Center in Mississippi have shown that plants can also act as effective filters. Former NASA scientist Bill C. Wolverton, Ph.D., has spent the past twenty-five years studying the ability of plants to clear volatile organic chemicals from indoor air. Wolverton predicts that within twenty years plants will be governmentally mandated in new buildings as a matter of public health.

According to the EPA, the most plentiful of the organic chemicals in the average indoor environment is formaldehyde. It is released from a host of household furnishings, including synthetic carpeting, particleboard (used to make bookcases, desks, and tables), foam insulation, upholstery, curtains, and even so-called air fresheners. Common house plants such as chrysanthemums, striped dracaena, dwarf date palms, and especially Boston ferns are excellent filters for removing formaldehyde. Spider plants are also effective in removing carbon monoxide; areca palms are best at filtering xylene, the second-most-prevalent indoor organic chemical; and English ivy is good for filtering benzene, ranked third on the EPA's list. Aloe vera, philodendron, pothos, and ficus were also found to reduce levels of organic chemicals.

The Foliage for Clean Air Council, a communications clearinghouse for information on the use of foliage to improve indoor air quality, recommends a minimum of two plants per 100 square feet of floor space in an average home with eight- to ten-foot ceilings.

Plants can help improve indoor air as oxygenators, filters, and humidifiers.

PREVENTION

Prevention of indoor air pollution involves eliminating pollutants at the source. Doctors who specialize in environmental medicine and some allergists can do skin and blood tests to help you identify pollutants to which you are particularly sensitive or allergic. These doctors are not always easy to find, nor are the tests always definitive, but they can help. With the use of environmentally sensitive architectural principles, a healthier home can be created. A major preventive strategy is the use of interior materials that emit no pollutants. Natural products such as wood, cotton, and metals are preferable to the lower-cost synthetic materials such as particleboard, fiberboard, polyester, and plastics.

Choosing to forgo a fireplace or wood-burning stove would be helpful, as would using a high-efficiency furnace with a sealed combustion unit to vent exhaust gases to the outside. Switch to nontoxic cleaning substances, including ordinary soap, vinegar, zephiran, and Air Therapy (you can find a listing of such cleaners in *Nontoxic, Natural, & Earthwise,* by Debra Lynn Dadd). Smoking should be relegated to the outdoors or to a well-ventilated enclosed space. If radon levels exceed the acceptable EPA standard of 4 picoCuries per liter of air, radon control measures should be implemented. Formaldehyde from insulation can be eliminated by using the substitutes of cellulose and white fiberglass insulation.

HUMIDIFICATION

According to Dr. Marshall Plaut, chief of the asthma and allergy branch at the National Institute of Allergy and Infectious Diseases (part of NIH), "Dry air triggers asthma and nasal congestion." I too have been convinced for quite some time that dry air, and especially cold and dry air, is a major contributor to sinusitis and chronic bronchitis. As a chronic irritant to the sensitive nasal mucous membrane, dry air can also contribute to a greater susceptibility to allergies. Studies on patients with allergic rhinitis have shown that warm, moist air can improve nasal congestion and other allergy symptoms.

Optimum indoor air quality requires air containing between 35 and 45 percent relative humidity. Moisture provided by room humidifiers can greatly benefit anyone with a respiratory condition. These humidifiers are most helpful in the winter (heavy "sinus season" runs from November through March), even in humid, cold-weather climates, because most heating systems dry the indoor air considerably.

Room humidifiers, also called tabletop models, have sufficient capacity to humidify a medium- to large-size room. Each type has some drawbacks. Ultrasonic models can emit an irritating white dust. So can cool mist models, which require the use of distilled water or an expensive demineralization cartridge, unless you have very soft water. Steam-mist models, also called vaporizers, can scald if you get too close to the mist they produce or if you tip them over by accident. Evaporative models, the most prevalent type, can become a breeding ground for bacteria. The warm-mist units are my first choice. They produce a mist just slightly warmer than room air, use tap water, require no filter, and they're able to kill bacteria. Their only downfall may be that they use more electricity than the other types. I've been quite pleased with the performance of the Bionaire Clear Mist 5 (CMP-5), a warm-mist unit that I have used for the past two winter seasons. The tabletop humidifiers can cost from $30 to $120.

The larger humidifiers, called consoles, can humidify an average-size house, cost from $100 to $200, and are all the evaporative type. Although I've had no personal experience with these, I know that *Consumer Reports* has given a high rating to the Bionaire W-6S, as well as to the Toastmaster 3435 and Emerson HD850.

Central or in-duct humidifiers, those that attach to the furnace, are more convenient but often do not humidify an individual room as well as a portable humidifier can when the door to the room is closed. The major problem with central humidifiers is that most of them are the reservoir type, with a tray of standing water that breeds mold and bacteria. I recommend the flow-through type of central humidifier, e.g. Aprilaire or General, which eliminates the stagnant water problem and is easy to maintain. Depending on the model, size of your home, and installation, this humidifier would probably cost about $250 to $650.

Humidifiers are not the only option for moisturizing your home. The installation of waterfalls, indoor spas, and swimming pools will all add a lot of moisture to the house, but, of course, they are expensive to install and maintain. It might surprise you to learn that even the moisture from human breath and sweat, along with that from cooking, baths, showers, and plants, adds significantly to a home's humidity. If your bedroom is dry, hang a wet towel on a hanger in the room.

If you rarely suffer jolts of static electricity when you touch metal objects such as doorknobs, then the air in your home is probably humid enough. For a more precise test, you'll need a hygrometer. You can find these humidity measuring devices at most hardware stores. The one I've been using is the Bionaire "Climate Check," a digital device that measures both temperature and humidity.

Chapter 8

PHYSICAL HEALTH

After almost twenty-five years as a physician, it has become quite clear to me that for anyone experiencing physical discomfort, life is not much fun. I am assuming that the majority of you have one or more of the chronic respiratory diseases. There is probably a small percentage of readers suffering from something other than a respiratory ailment and an even smaller group who feel fine physically but are interested in experiencing a greater degree of health. I am making an educated guess that most of you would not have gone to the trouble of buying and reading this book if you do not have at least one very uncomfortable physical symptom that has not been relieved with the treatment you've been using. The focus of holistic medicine is on restoring health to the whole person—body, mind, and spirit—and on addressing the causes of dis-ease. But I have found that it's extremely difficult for individuals to improve their mental or spiritual health if their bodies are not functioning properly and they're in constant pain, having trouble breathing, or have no energy.

The holistic approach to physical fitness will allow you to develop far greater awareness and appreciation for your body. You will learn how to listen to the messages your body is communicating on a daily basis and allow your body to heal itself. Through this heightened sensitivity you will develop more vitality and energy, a more powerful immune system, and the ability to perform personally challenging physical feats. But your first order of physical "business" is "to get rid of this damn ____!"

SYMPTOM TREATMENT

I would recommend beginning the Sinus Survival Program with an aggressive approach to treating the symptoms of your sinusitis, allergies, asthma, bronchitis, or any other chronic condition. This includes consulting with your physician and making sure that you have treated your ailment with the best methods that conventional medicine has to offer, even if they provide only symptomatic relief. However, it is essential that you try to determine if the benefits of that treatment, such as drugs and surgery, outweigh the liabilities. As I've previously mentioned, in the case of chronic sinusitis, the continued use of antibiotics (more than three courses within a six-month period) is potentially more of a detriment than an asset. If you have been taking multiple antibiotics for months or years, follow the recommendations in this chapter and the next, "Candida." Together they will provide you with a natural, safe, and effective alternative to the chronic use of antibiotics, while you undo the damage done by the antibiotics. I realize that it might sound like too great a risk, but stopping antibiotics is invariably the first step most of my patients must take before they can cure chronic sinusitis.

As you begin this physical approach to treating your symptoms, remember the images that I've mentioned earlier in the book—the fine sandpaper abrading the sensitive mucous membranes, or the onslaught of pollutants assaulting the lining of the entire respiratory tract with every breath, 23,000 times a day. It is the *healing of this chronically irritated and inflamed mucous membrane that should now become the object of your treatment plan*. This dysfunctional and weakened membrane is a primary cause of most of your symptoms. Suppose you now replace that earlier image of assaulting with one of gently caressing and bathing that delicate mucosa with perfectly fresh, clean, warm, and moist air, with every breath you take. This healing vision can be expanded in any way you'd like. But it is important to keep it in mind, since it will help to keep you on the right track as you choose different treatment options. For instance, if your nose is really stuffed up, you might opt for soothing steam rather than blast your already inflamed membranes with a decongestant nasal spray. It works almost as quickly; it's just not quite as convenient. But most important, it heals rather than harms as it treats your symptoms. Decongestants, expectorants, cough suppressants, analgesics, nasal irrigation, saline sprays, pure drinking water, negative-ion generators, humidifiers, air duct cleaning, and plants are all methods for treating symptoms that have already been described. From that list, regular irrigation, the saline spray, and the use of an ionizer and humidifier at work and in your bedroom are probably the most effective measures for both treating symptoms and healing the mucous membranes. Antibiotics are fine if you have only one or two infections per year, but they are by no means mandatory in treating a sinus infection.

As you begin the Sinus Survival Program, it is often helpful to rate each of your symptoms on a scale of 1 to 10, with 1 being an almost incapacitating symptom and 10 being perfectly normal (no symptom). You can use the "Symptom Chart" (pp. 129–30) and rate yourself at the end of each week. It provides you with both an objective (most of the symptoms can be measured objectively—you can either see, hear, or feel them) and subjective (especially energy level) means of monitoring your progress. You don't need anyone else or an X-ray or lab test to tell you how well you're doing.

The foundation of the physical aspect of holistic medical treatment is to love and nurture your body with safe and gentle therapies. You should have a much better idea of how to do that, especially for your respiratory tract, after reading this chapter.

Symptom Chart

Began Sinus Survival Program on _____
Rate Symptoms from 1 (worst) to 10 (best = normal)

SYMPTOM	BEGIN _____ (date)	END WEEK 1	END WEEK 2	END WEEK 3	END WEEK 4	END WEEK 5	END WEEK 6	END WEEK 7	END WEEK 8	END WEEK 9	END WEEK 10	END WEEK 11	END WEEK 12
Head Congestion (fullness)													
Nasal Congestion (stuffy nose)													
Postnasal Drip													
Headache													
Yellow/Green Mucus (from nose)													
Yellow/Green Mucus (back of throat)													
Sneezing													
Itching: Nose, Throat													
Ear Congestion (ears plugged up)													
Sore Throat													
Swollen Glands (in neck)													
Cough—dry													

SYMPTOM	BEGIN ___ (date)	END WEEK 1	END WEEK 2	END WEEK 3	END WEEK 4	END WEEK 5	END WEEK 6	END WEEK 7	END WEEK 8	END WEEK 9	END WEEK 10	END WEEK 11	END WEEK
Cough—wet/mucusy													
Shortness of Breath													
Wheezing													
Fatigue (rate energy level)													
Avg # of hrs sleep													
Other Symptoms:													
Medications: (Pharmaceutical Drugs) (use a "√" if still taking drug)													

DIET

"We are what we eat." I have heard that saying many times, but it never made much of an impact until I began changing my diet in the process of treating my own chronic sinusitis. I am now convinced that most chronic medical conditions can be helped significantly by a healthy diet. With specific regard to the respiratory tract, the change I recommend most is to avoid milk and dairy products. They tend to increase and thicken mucus secretions. If you would like to compensate for the loss of calcium in your own or your child's diet, the following foods are especially rich in calcium: broccoli, kale, sesame seeds and sesame seed butter, tofu, sea vegetables, and soy cheese. You can also buy a liquid calcium and magnesium combination at most health-food stores. An adequate daily dose for an adult female is 1,200 mg of calcium and 500 to 600 mg of magnesium.

Sugar should also be avoided, especially if you suspect that candida is contributing to your sinusitis. A nutritionist once asked me, "Would you fill the gas tank of your car with sand?" She felt that filling your body with sugar is equally destructive. Yet the average American eats or drinks the equivalent of 41 teaspoons of sugar every day! It seems to be in almost everything, from nearly all breakfast cereals to table salt. Sugar not only has no nutritional value, it is also harmful. There is scientific evidence that it weakens the immune system, making us more susceptible to both infection and allergy.

Caffeine is a drug to which most Americans are addicted. The average person drinks two and a half cups of coffee a day. Coffee has roughly three times the caffeine of tea. Caffeine is a stimulant that races our engines for a few hours, only to leave us with a greater sense of fatigue when the effect wears off. The quick fix for this state of low energy is usually to drink another cup of coffee or tea or another bottle of caffeine-rich soda pop. Your entire body suffers as a result of being on a perpetual "roller coaster."

The evidence seems to indicate that limiting ourselves to one or two cups of coffee per day would be relatively safe. However, the majority of us drink more than that, and are therefore at higher risk for a variety of health problems. The following table was prepared by Robert A. Anderson, M.D., a family physician and author of *Wellness Medicine*.

In addition to the "beneficial effects" listed by Dr. Anderson, caffeine in low to moderate doses (less than 200 mg, or one or two cups of coffee) has been scientifically shown to make you

Table 8-1

Caffeine

Use
More than 50% of Americans drink coffee daily. Average caffeine daily consumption by those who drink is 400 mg/day.

Hazardous Effects

Blood Pressure
200–400 mg (1-$\frac{1}{2}$ to 2-$\frac{1}{2}$ cups of coffee) increases adrenaline 200%, noradrenaline 75%, renin 60%, systolic blood pressure 14mmHg, diastolic blood pressure 10mmHg, and respiratory rate 20%.

Cancer
Some (not all) reports relate coffee to a higher incidence of pancreatic cancer; mutagens have been found in coffee.

Cardiac effects
Contributes to heart rhythm disturbances. Four or more cups of coffee/day (decaf or not) increases men's rate of heart disease 30% and women's 60%.

Central nervous system
Stimulates the central nervous system.

Circulation
Causes local vasoconstriction by blocking adenosine release; causes dizziness.

Clotting
Decreases platelet stickiness.

Degenerative disease and free radicals
Increases adrenaline; adrenaline metabolites increase free radicals and risks of degenerative diseases.

Gastrointestinal effects
Stimulates gastric acid secretion.

Interaction with drugs
Interacts and/or competes with prescription drugs.

Muscular effects
Is a major factor in restless legs syndrome; contributes to muscle tension syndromes by promoting calcium loss from muscle cells.

Osteoporosis
Contributes to osteoporosis by increasing calcium loss; one cup of coffee raises calcium requirements 30–50 mg.

Pain
Coffee contains a narcotic antagonist and may decrease pain tolerance.

Pregnancy
May contribute to certain problems in pregnancy.

Psychoactive effects
Causes anxiety and irritability; very large amounts can precipitate psychosis and acute schizophrenia; can precipitate agoraphobia in susceptible persons; affects adenosine and beta-adrenergic receptors causing euphoria, tolerance, dependence, addiction, and symptoms of physical withdrawal.

Sleep
Caffeine reduces the depth of sleep.

Urinary tract
Increases urinary frequency.

BENEFICIAL EFFECTS
Caffeine and coffee act as a stimulant, can lengthen sleep latency, thus keeping people awake.

think faster, perform certain mental tasks better, and improve both alertness and mood.

Prominent cancer researcher John Weisburger, director emeritus of the American Health Foundation, believes that tea is an effective antioxidant (see p. 142), and that the chemicals in tea may help counteract carcinogens in food, especially in grilled, fried, and broiled meat. Researchers at the National Institute of Nutrition in Rome found that black and green tea raise antioxidant activity in the blood by 40 to 50 percent. Other studies have found that black and green tea can reduce the risk of fatal heart disease and some cancers. These teas can be found in most health food stores and some supermarkets.

Table 8-2

Caffeine Amounts (mg)

COFFEE, 5-OUNCE CUP
Decaffeinated instant: 2
Decaffeinated brewed: 2–5
Instant: 40–108
Percolated: 64–124
Drip: 110–150

TEA, 5-OUNCE CUP
Bag, brewed for five minutes: 20–50
Bag, brewed for one minute: 9–33
Loose, black, five-minute brew: 20–85
Loose, green, five-minute brew: 15–80
Iced: 22 to 36

SOFT DRINKS, 12-OUNCE GLASS
Cola: 44–46

CHOCOLATE
Cocoa, 5-ounce cup: 4–6
Milk chocolate, 1 ounce: 3–6
Bittersweet chocolate, 1 ounce: 25–35

Reactions to caffeine vary widely from person to person and stem in part from genetic differences in the way the body metabolizes it. Smoking reduces the effect of caffeine, while pregnancy and birth control pills can enhance it.

The best way to break caffeine addiction is to do it very *gradually,* over a week, substituting noncaffeinated beverages such as herb tea or a roasted-grain beverage. Be aware of the possible withdrawal symptoms of headache, nervousness, and irritability.

I'm sure that most of you are familiar with the recommendation to decrease your consumption of red meat and egg yolks. Both are significant sources of cholesterol, which is a major contributor to heart disease. Recent research by the USDA suggests that a low-fat diet may also strengthen your immune system.

Alcohol should be consumed only in moderate amounts (two to three beers, or one cocktail, or a glass of wine per day). Studies have shown that complete abstainers from alcohol have a slightly shorter life expectancy than those who drink in moderate amounts. However, if candidiasis is aggravating your chronic sinusitis, don't drink any alcohol for at least three months during treatment. Since sugar and alcohol seem to be major dietary contributors to the problem of candida, it is not difficult to understand how the typical American diet has encouraged this widespread infection.

Although most people drink and smoke to feel better, there is evidence that both alcohol and nicotine significantly contribute to feelings of depression, loneliness, restlessness, and boredom. Based on research studies from the National Center for Health Statistics, almost 40 million Americans experienced at least one of those unpleasant states during the two weeks before being interviewed. Lonely adults were 60 to 70 percent more likely to smoke, and depressed adults were 40 to 50 percent more likely to light up. The moodiest men were three times as likely to be heavy drinkers (three or more drinks a day).

Try to decrease your consumption of food additives. These include chemical preservatives (such as BHA, BHT, sodium nitrite, and sulfites), artificial colors, and artificial sweeteners (including saccharin, aspartame [NutraSweet], and cyclamates). Almost every one of these additives has been shown to have a potential health risk.

Perhaps our biggest problem with food is our enormous American appetite. We eat about 40 percent more calories than we need, and obesity (weighing 20 percent above ideal body weight) has become epidemic. A massive nine-year U.S. study on caloric intake involving two dozen laboratories, sixty government and university researchers, and 24,000 rats and mice is currently in its eighth year. The results of restricting caloric intake by 40 percent have had a dramatic impact on increasing longevity. The most prominent advocate of human caloric restriction is Roy L. Wolford, M.D., an immunologist at the University of California at Los Angeles, who has raised some of the world's oldest mice using caloric restriction. His findings are described in his books *Maximum Lifespan* and *The 120-Year Diet.*

Our society has chosen food as its greatest treat, and unfortunately, the most highly prized foods not only have no nutritional value but ultimately can make us sick. Now that I have eliminated many of your life's greatest pleasures—ice cream, soda pop, sugar, coffee, and alcohol—as well as 40 percent of your calories, I hope you are still with me. I'm sorry. I can tell you, though, that when I stopped eating my evening bowl of ice cream nearly eight years ago, I thought it would be a lot more difficult than it turned out to be. What happens is that shortly after making these dietary changes, you will begin to appreciate new rewards: more energy, less mucus, fewer pounds, and a great feeling of accomplishment that comes from applying self-discipline toward doing something beneficial for yourself. Remember, too, that these are just recommendations, not commandments. My own guideline on this subject is "Everything in moderation, including moderation." I do believe, however, that if you are miserable with sick sinuses you should try to adhere as closely as possible to these suggestions. Try to make at least a three-month commitment to this diet.

A *healthy diet* is generally rich in fruits, fresh vegetables, whole grains (e.g., brown rice, bulgur, wheat, oats, amaranth, millet, quinoa, barley, and couscous, legumes, and fiber—abundant in bran cereals, beans, apricots, and prunes). Raw foods are usually better than cooked. Good sources of protein are nuts, seeds, fish, turkey, chicken, and the soybean products tofu and tempeh. The foods that most strengthen the immune system are also highly beneficial to those whose sinus condition is caused by nasal allergies; these are garlic, onions, citrus fruits, and horseradish.

In January 1992, the U.S. Department of Agriculture unveiled a new shape for the ideal American diet: a pyramid built on a base of grains (see Figure 8-1).

This is a very brief discussion of nutrition. Classes on the subject or consultation with a nutritionist would help you tailor a healthy diet to your personal tastes. Two books often recom-

Food Guide Pyramid

A Guide to Daily Food Choices

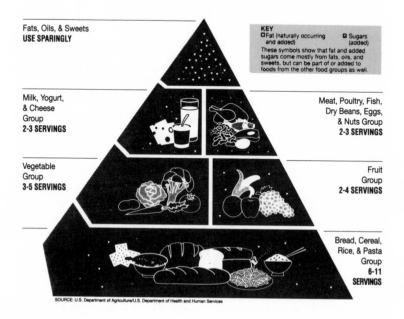

Fats, Oils, & Sweets
USE SPARINGLY

KEY
▢ Fat (naturally occurring   ▨ Sugars
and added)   (added)
These symbols show that fat and added sugars come mostly from fats, oils, and sweets, but can be part of or added to foods from the other food groups as well.

Milk, Yogurt, & Cheese Group
2-3 SERVINGS

Meat, Poultry, Fish, Dry Beans, Eggs, & Nuts Group
2-3 SERVINGS

Vegetable Group
3-5 SERVINGS

Fruit Group
2-4 SERVINGS

Bread, Cereal, Rice, & Pasta Group
6-11 SERVINGS

SOURCE: U.S. Department of Agriculture/U.S. Department of Health and Human Services

mended by nutritionists are *Food Is Your Best Medicine* by Henry G. Bieler, M.D., and *Vibrant Health from Your Kitchen* by Bernard Jensen, N.D..

If you have followed the preceding recommendations without a noticeable improvement in your condition. I suggest eliminating from your diet for at least three weeks the foods that most commonly produce the allergic reactions that might cause chronic sinusitis, allergies, and asthma: cow's milk and all dairy products, wheat or any grain, chocolate, corn, white sugar, soy, yeast (brewer's and baker's), oranges, tomatoes, bell peppers, white potatoes, eggs, fish, shellfish, cocoa, onions, nuts, garlic, peanuts, black pepper, red meat, aspirin, artificial food coloring, coffee, black tea, beer, wine, and champagne. I realize how difficult this can be, but it only need be for three weeks. After that, begin to reintroduce each of these foods into your diet at the rate of one every three days. Pay attention to your body and note any new symptoms such as headache, nausea, diarrhea, gas, or mental "fog." It then should be obvious to you which food, if any, causes your body to react. If you suspect food sensitivities, or suffer from hypoglycemia or chronic fatigue, the book *High Energy* by Rob Krakovitz, M.D., is an excellent resource.

I wish there were some way to make dietary change both simple and easy. If there were, I am sure it wouldn't have taken so many years for my family's diet to have reached the healthy point it has—and even that was with the added impetus of my daughter Carin's wish to be a vegetarian. If there is a good health-food store not too far from your home, try to shop there. The salespeople are usually very helpful. Many supermarkets now have health-food sections. Take a few extra minutes on your next trip to see what looks good. Be a little adventuresome, but do try to implement change gradually. This transition should not be made in two weeks. Those who take their time have a much greater chance of maintaining their healthy diet. Although there are many powerful therapeutic measures to help your nose, sinuses, and lungs, few are more valuable than eating only food that is nourishing and non-allergenic to your body.

WATER

Water has been called our most essential nutrient. Regular water drinking might be the simplest, least expensive self-help measure for the maintenance of good health.

The percentage of water in a human body varies from 60 to 80 percent. At birth, a baby's body is about 80 percent water, and the average adult's body is between 60 and 70 percent. Every bodily function occurs through the medium of water. Water helps to cleanse the blood by removing wastes through the kidneys; it is vital to digestion and metabolism; it is crucial to nerve impulse conduction; it carries nutrients and oxygen to the cells through the blood; it helps to regulate our body temperature through perspiration; it lubricates our joints; and as I have already mentioned, the respiratory tract needs it to lubricate the mucous membrane. The sinuses drain more easily when you are well hydrated and their mucous membrane is more resistant to infection.

Unfortunately, many Americans are chronically dehydrated. This condition can impair every aspect of the body's normal functioning, resulting in reduced blood volume with less oxygen and nutrients provided to all muscles and organs, excess body fat, poor muscle tone and size, decreased digestive efficiency (constipation), increased toxicity in the body, joint and muscle soreness (especially after exercise), and water retention (the body retains water to compensate for the shortage). This is why proper water intake is important for weight loss. In general, we need to drink more water than our thirst calls for.

A healthy but sedentary adult weighing 160 pounds should drink about ten 8-ounce glasses of water a day (one-half ounce per pound of body weight); an active, athletic person of the same weight should drink thirteen to fourteen 8-ounce glasses a day (two-thirds ounce per pound). Try to spread your intake throughout the day (it's best to drink between meals), and don't drink more than four glasses in any given hour. Don't substitute beer, coffee, tea, soft drinks, or processed fruit juice for pure water. Although they all contain water, they also have other ingredients that can negate the positive effect of water. Herbal tea, natural fruit juices (without sugar and diluted 50 percent with water), and some soups (low salt, no sugar, the clearer and thinner the better) can substitute for a portion of your daily water requirement. Often overlooked is the fact that we also obtain water by absorbing it through our skin while bathing and showering.

Water quality is so variable in the United States that it is impossible to generalize about whether you should drink tap, bottled, or filtered water. I don't recommend distilled water for drinking because it doesn't provide the necessary minerals. In some communities the water is so pure they don't even need to treat it; other sources contain high levels of lead and radon, the two worst contaminants. Radon can cause cancer, and lead can impair the development of brain cells in children. Nationwide, drinking water is responsible for 20 percent of all lead contamination. Adverse effects from lead can occur at very low levels. Early symptoms of lead poisoning—such as nervousness, irritability, headaches, fatigue, muscular problems, constipation, and indigestion—are hard to pinpoint as lead-related. One way to reduce the risk of lead poisoning is to run your tap in the morning to flush out the contaminated water. Avoid drinking tap water that has been sitting in the plumbing for a few hours, and don't cook with or drink water from the hot-water tap because hot water can dissolve lead more quickly. Unfortunately, you can't depend on the local government to protect you from water pollution. According to Gene Rosov, president of WaterTest Corporation, the nation's largest independent drinking-water testing laboratory, "The majority of the health-related risks that are present in drinking water are a result of the contamination added *after* the water leaves the treatment and distribution plant." This means that it would be a good idea to have the water at your tap tested, regardless of your local water utility's claims about water quality. Call your health department for a referral for testing. Reverse-osmosis filters appear to be the most effective home water-filtering systems presently available. But there are also some distillation and carbon filters that are able to significantly reduce lead in water. There are carafe-style filters for the kitchen faucet that cost about $25, under-the-sink models for $400, and point-of-entry units that purify the water as it enters the house. These can cost as much as $1,250.

It is a fact of life in America today that we can never know for certain whether what we drink or eat is completely safe. Do the best you can. Remember to drink more water and to make it convenient (keep a water container in your car and at your desk while working). Don't wait until you're thirsty to drink, and most important, be sure that there's always a bathroom nearby.

HYDROTHERAPY

Other than drinking, irrigating, moistening, bathing, or soaking in it, I've found that water can be therapeutic by virtue of its temperature. While taking a shower, increase the temperature as much as you are able to tolerate and allow this hot water to strike your face, especially the area around your nose and sinuses. To prolong your tolerance you can move your face from side to side or in a circular motion. If you are congested or have a sinus infection, this technique will help relieve the congestion and allow the sinuses to drain.

Both as a therapeutic and preventive measure that can strengthen the immune system, I also recommend turning off the hot water completely and allowing the cold water to strike your mid-chest for about a minute. I learned this technique from Dr. Steve Morris, a naturopathic physician, in 1989. He explained that it is a commonly prescribed hydrotherapeutic technique in naturopathic medicine for stimulating the thymus gland—an important component of the immune system located in your chest cavity directly under the sternum (breastbone). I've been practicing this technique routinely ever since, just before I finish showering. I can't be certain what it's doing for my thymus, but it definitely stimulates the rest of my body!

VITAMINS, HERBS, SUPPLEMENTS, AND ANTIOXIDANTS

In case you hadn't noticed, life in urban America can be extremely stressful. Almost daily we are exposed to chemical stress, emotional stress, and infection. Each type of stress has numerous sources. Chemical stress, for example, may come from polluted air, polluted water, food pesticides, insecticides, heavy metals, or, worst of all, radioactive wastes. More than ever, we are exposed to a myriad of foreign chemicals, both commercially synthesized and naturally occurring in our environment. The 1989 Kellogg Report stated that 1,000 newly synthesized compounds are introduced each year, which amounts to three new chemicals a day. The current number of foreign chemicals (called xenobiotics) now totals around 100,000 and includes drugs, pesticides, industrial chemicals, food additives and preservatives, and environmental pollutants. Toxic chemicals easily find their way into our body through the air we breathe, the food we eat, and the water we drink. We also ingest foreign chemicals when taking medicinal or illicit drugs, or when using alcohol or tobacco.

Although the body is designed to eliminate toxins, it cannot always handle the overload present in today's environment. Unfortunately, we still know very little about the magnitude of the harmful effects caused by our continual exposure to these chemicals. In this book, you're learning about some of these toxic effects on the respiratory tract. There are several studies that reveal a strong correlation between high exposure to air pollutants and pesticides and contracting cancer. David Abbey, Ph.D., a professor of biostatistics at Loma Linda University, found that women living in the Los Angeles area have a 37 percent greater risk of developing *all forms of cancer* as a result of high exposure to particulates than women who live in cleaner air environments. His studies also revealed a 125 percent higher risk for both men and women of getting lung cancer from high levels of ozone pollution.

We are learning that all stressors—chemical, emotional, and infectious—harm us by weakening our immune systems with highly toxic molecules called free radicals. According to Deepak Chopra, M.D., author of *Quantum Healing: Exploring the Frontiers of Mind/Body Medicine* and *Ageless Body, Timeless Mind,* free radicals are the "metabolic end-products in the body of environmental pollution, food toxins, carcinogens, and emotional toxins."

Medical research has already implicated free radicals as causative factors in many diseases (e.g., arthritis, mental disorders, and heart disease), as well as in susceptibility to infection and in the process of aging. In fact, over the past thirty years, research has revealed a common factor in every degenerative disease of our time: cell damage as a result of free radicals. Denham Harman, M.D., of the University of Nebraska says, "Today it seems very likely that the assumption that there is a basic cause of aging is correct and that the sum of deleterious free radical reactions going on continuously throughout the cells and tissues is the aging process or a major contribution to it."

Free radicals are responsible for most cellular damage. Fortunately, our bodies manufacture antioxidant enzymes within the cells for protection against free radicals, and also employ antioxidant nutrients (e.g., vitamin A [beta-carotene], vitamin E, and vitamin C) supplied by our diet. As long as there is an adequate supply of oxygen, water, antioxidant nutrients, and enzymes in the body, cell damage is minimized. When any one of these is deficient, cell damage is accelerated, as in the process of aging and in disease. Through their critical role in helping to prevent disease, *vitamins, acting as antioxidants, can offer considerable help to our body's immune system.*

When disease, including any of the chronic respiratory diseases, is present, the cells are overrun with an excess of free radicals and the immune system cannot maintain its protective shield. This occurs when stress lowers our body's production of antioxidant enzymes to a level less than our needs. Unfortunately, city living makes it difficult to avoid most of our stressors. It is a wonder that the majority of us are free of a chronic disease. For those who have not been as fortunate, and for anyone interested in strengthening their body's natural defenses, practicing preventive medicine, or experiencing a greater degree of physical health, the following recommendations for vitamins, herbs, and nutritional supplements will help.

Vitamin C

In 1970 the distinguished chemist and Nobel Prize winner Linus Pauling turned his attention to the benefits of megadoses of vitamin C in the prevention and treatment of colds. The verification of his findings by other researchers has been complicated primarily by the great variability in the dosages and types of vitamin C that have been used. In my experience, vitamin C has been extremely effective in the treatment and prevention of both colds and sinus infections. In that colds are the most common cause of acute sinusitis, their prevention is good preventive medicine for sinusitis. In addition to its antioxidant properties, vitamin C is essential to the manufacture of collagen, the main supportive protein of skin, tendon, bone, cartilage, and connective tissue; has an anti-inflammatory effect, especially in some autoimmune diseases such as lupus and rheumatoid arthritis; facilitates the absorption of dietary iron; enhances the immune response and white blood cell activity; and, in conjunction with vitamin E, strengthens arterial walls. In a recent study conducted by researchers from the USDA and National Institute on Aging, vitamin C was shown to provide greater protection against cholesterol buildup (by raising HDL—the "good" cholesterol) and reduce the risk of heart disease. Another study suggests that it can help prevent chronic bronchitis.

The average daily dose for cold prevention is 3,000 milligrams (mg). If you already have a cold or sinus infection, I recommend as much as 15,000 mg a day. Take this amount in divided dosages, either 5,000 mg three times a day with meals (to avoid stomach upset, it is best to take most vitamins with food) or 2,000 to 3,000 mg every two to three hours, preferably in a powdered form as ascorbate. This is much more easily absorbed and more potent than ascorbic acid—the more common form of vitamin C found in fruits, vegetables, and most commercial brands of vitamin C. You can also take time-released vitamin C capsules or tablets that are assimilated over twelve hours. Most other vitamin C tablets last for only six to eight hours. This high dosage for colds and sinus infections should be maintained for several days, or until your symptoms begin to improve. Taper off very gradually over the next two weeks to get back down to the usual daily dose of 3,000 mg. Dr. Pauling's prescription: at the first sign of a cold, take 1,000 mg or more of vitamin C every hour during the waking hours. Possible side effects of dosages above 3,000 mg are diarrhea, bowel gas, and cramps. But these symptoms are more likely to occur with the pure ascorbic acid form of vitamin C. If you experience these symptoms, cut back on your next dose by 1,000 mg. A less common side effect is the development of kidney stones. This can usually be prevented by drinking the recommended daily amount of water or by taking 75 mg of vitamin B_6 a day.

Another method for taking vitamin C, called titrating to bowel tolerance, was developed by Robert Cathcart, M.D. Cathcart has treated over 9,000 patients with large doses of ascorbic acid, some as great as 100,000 mg a day. He believes the maximum relief of symptoms is obtained at a point just short of the amount that produces diarrhea. According to Dr. Cathcart, the amount of vitamin C that can be taken orally without causing diarrhea when a person is ill might be as much as ten times the amount he or she would tolerate if well. Using this method, he claims success treating a host of viral infections, including colds, influenza, mononucleosis, and viral pneumonia; environmental and food allergies; cancer; rheumatoid arthritis; hepatitis; and yeast infections.

There is quite a variation in the strength of different brands of vitamin C. For instance, 1,000 mg of ascorbate is better absorbed than 1,000 mg of ascorbic acid. Once ascorbic acid is absorbed into our bloodstream, it reacts with many minerals, such as sodium, calcium, magnesium, and zinc, to form ascorbates. It is in this form, as ascorbates, that vitamin C enters the trillions of cells in our bodies. The commercial brands of C that I recommend are any form of Ester C (some studies indicate it may be the most potent form of C); Alacer Super Gram II timed release or the powder Emergen-C; Ethical Nutrients esterified polyascorbate; and Nature's Plus Ascorbate C. Taking vitamin C in ascorbate powder is the most effective way to enhance absorption.

Vitamin C, as an antioxidant, is a free-radical scavenger. Our bodies can use a lot more of it when we are under stress. Use your own discretion in varying your dosage, depending on the degree of stress you think you have experienced that day. If it was a high air pollution day or if you had a rough time at work, take more than the 3,000 mg. The same recommendation holds true for all of the other vitamins and herbs I will mention in the following sections. Vitamin C and all of the other vitamins and herbs are more effective if eaten in the natural form of food rather than taken in pill or powder forms. The foods highest in vitamin C are red chili peppers, red sweet peppers, green sweet peppers, kale, parsley, collard greens, turnip greens, mustard greens, broccoli, brussels sprouts, cauliflower, guavas, oranges, cantaloupe, and strawberries. Their vitamin C content is higher when eaten raw.

Linus Pauling died in 1994 at the age of ninety-three of prostate cancer. He reportedly took 10,000 mg of vitamin C every day.

Vitamin A and Beta-Carotene

Most vitamin A comes from its precursor, beta-carotene, which is converted to the vitamin form in the gastrointestinal tract. Beta-carotene is a substance in carotenoids, which are usually found in yellow, orange, or red foods. Listed in roughly descending order of vitamin A content, these include carrots, sweet potatoes, yams, kale, spinach, mangoes, winter squash, cantaloupe, apricots, broccoli, romaine lettuce, asparagus, tomatoes, nectarines, peaches, and papayas. Vitamin A itself can be obtained directly from consumption of cod liver oil, liver, kidney, eggs, and dairy products.

Vitamin A helps to maintain the integrity of mucous membranes, is required for growth and repair of cells, is necessary for protein metabolism, protects night vision, and protects against cancer. Beta-carotene has been shown to have an effect as an anticancer nutrient—a discovery made by Japanese researchers more than twenty years ago. It is also a powerful antioxidant and a potent immunostimulator. In recent research conducted by Charles Hennekens, M.D., of Harvard Medical School, beta-carotene was found to reduce dramatically (by 50 percent) strokes and heart attacks in people who already have cardiovascular disease. Adequate beta-carotene in the diet should supply the vitamin A you need, but vitamin A deficiency in the United States is not uncommon. According to a survey by the U.S. Department of Health, Education, and Welfare, about 60 percent of women and 50 percent of men have intakes below the standard set for good nutrition. Pure vitamin A can be toxic to the liver in prolonged dosages greater than 50,000 I.U. (international units) a day, but beta-carotene is not. The only side effect of high doses of beta-carotene is yellowing skin, which is not dangerous and disappears when levels are reduced. For sinus infections it is recommended that you take beta-carotene at 50,000 I.U. two times a day. After the acute infection has been resolved, this dosage can be cut at least in half and continued indefinitely.

Vitamin E

The specific functions of vitamin E are unclear. It has recently been recognized as an antioxidant and in some studies has been shown to raise levels of the desirable cholesterol, HDL. According to Nabil Elsayed, Ph.D., a professor of public health at UCLA, "You will definitely improve your chances of resisting smog if you increase your vitamin E intake." He believes that vitamin E can significantly reduce lung damage from ozone. Another recent study indicates that E helps to prevent asthma. For people with sinusitis, allergies, asthma, and bronchitis, 400 I.U. of vitamin E daily are recommended, and should be taken as mixed tocopherols. When it is combined with selenium, vitamin E becomes twice as potent. This dosage need not be reduced as the symptoms of infection subside. Foods highest in vitamin E are crude and unrefined soybean oil and wheat germ oil, fresh wheat germ, whole grains, raw nuts (most varieties), and all green, leafy vegetables.

Multivitamins

There are many comparable multivitamins from which to choose. Make sure your choice has all of the B vitamins and is yeast-free. Take one daily whether you have any of the respiratory conditions or not, and in addition to the vitamin supplements A, C, and E.

Minerals

The two minerals that seem most effective in aiding the body's immune system are selenium and zinc. A recent article in the *Journal of the National Cancer Institute* said that men with lower levels of selenium in their blood were most likely to develop cancers of the lung, stomach, and pancreas. Low selenium levels might also be linked to bladder cancer and asthma. To treat symptomatic sinus infections I recommend either selenium citrate, aspartate, or picolinate in a dosage of 195 micrograms (mcg) daily; or selenium in a combination pill with vitamin E. Foods high in selenium are whole-wheat products, fish, whole grains, mushrooms, beans, garlic, and liver. Selenium can be toxic to the body, so don't maintain a daily dosage greater than 200 mcg for longer than two weeks. Then reduce it to a maintenance dosage between 100 to 150.

Zinc appears to be critical to the release of vitamin A from the liver and is vital to the process by which new cells are produced and protein metabolized for repair of body tissues. People with sinusitis should take 15 mg of zinc picolinate or oratate three times a day, but only when symptomatic. The foods highest in zinc are beef liver and the dark meat of turkey. The recommended maintenance dosage of zinc is 15 mg, which can be taken in your multivitamin.

Herbs, Botanicals, and Other Remedies

It has been estimated that nearly 25 percent of all pharmaceutical drugs are made from plants, herbs, leaves, bark, or roots. In September 1990, cancer researchers asked the Department of the Interior for federal protection for the Pacific yew, a tree found in the ancient forests of the Pacific Northwest whose bark provides a scarce new cancer-fighting drug. The fact that we are destroying global forests so rapidly, especially the rain forests, means that we are eliminating potentially life-saving drugs without even knowing it. Many species of plants are becoming extinct before botanists can determine their value. There are still a few human cultures remaining that depend almost entirely on naturally occurring vegetation for their medicines.

Onions; the herbs garlic, echinacea, and goldenseal; and bee propolis all seem to strengthen the immune system to such an extent that they might be called natural antibiotics. I recommend all of them to patients fighting a sinus infection or acute bronchitis. They can be taken in addition to a pharmaceutical antibiotic in the form of a capsule, liquid, or tea. Good reference books for medicinal herbs are *A Textbook of Natural Medicine* by Joseph Pizzorno, N.D., and *The Complete Botanical Prescriber* by John Sherman, N.D.

Garlic, a member of the lily family, is a perennial plant, cultivated around the world, that has been prescribed throughout history to treat a variety of ailments. Egyptians have been using it for almost 5,000 years, and the Chinese for at least 3,000 years. Hippocrates and Aristotle cited many therapeutic uses for garlic, including the relief of coughs, toothache, earache, dandruff, hypertension, atherosclerosis, diarrhea and dysentery, and vaginitis. It can be effective as an antibacterial, antiviral, antifungal, antihypertensive, and anti-inflammatory agent. At the National Cancer Institute garlic has recently shown promise in fighting stomach and colon cancer. Garlic is for the most part nontoxic, although it does cause bad breath. Many brands of processed garlic are available at health-food stores in pill, capsule, and liquid forms. Raw garlic is best, up to one clove per day.

Echinacea is at the top of the list of immunity-enhancing herbs. A perennial herb native to the American Midwest, it serves as an immunostimulator, wound healer, and anti-inflammatory, antiviral, antibacterial, and antineoplastic (cancer). It can be taken alone or in a liquid combination with goldenseal, in a dosage of forty drops three times a day. It also comes in capsules. Think of echinacea as you would an antibiotic. It must be taken regularly in order to have a therapeutic effect, but if taken beyond three weeks it is possible to build up a tolerance to its therapeutic effect. Naturopathic physician, Dr. Steve Morris grows some of the highest grade echinacea in America, on his farm near Seattle. He recommends to his patients that they take the herb daily until their symptoms are completely gone, and continue for another three to four days beyond that point.

Goldenseal is a perennial herb native to eastern North America and is cultivated in Oregon and Washington state. It is best known for its action in soothing inflammatory conditions of the respiratory, digestive, and genitourinary tracts caused by allergy or infection. It enhances the function of the mucous membranes. Goldenseal should not be taken by women who are pregnant or who plan a pregnancy in the near future. People with known or suspected hypoglycemia and ragweed pollen allergies might have an adverse reaction. I have seen only three patients who have been allergic to goldenseal. There is also considered to be a minimal risk to children and people over age fifty-five with the use of goldenseal, and it should not be taken in large quantities for extended periods of time. For treating an infection, you can take twenty to thirty drops three times a day.

Bee propolis is an extract from the bee's body (it is *not* bee pollen), and it comes in both liquid and capsules. The dosage is 500 mg three times a day. If you use the liquid form, follow the instructions on the bottle. Bee propolis appears to enhance immune function.

There are a growing number of products available containing the herb *ephedra,* a natural decongestant and bronchodilator, from which many of the pharmaceutical decongestants have been derived. Ephedra combined with herbal expectorants is an effective natural method of treating sinusitis, asthma, and allergy symptoms. There are a number of products available in health food stores containing ephedra in combination with other beneficial herbs. The Chinese herb Ma huang is also ephedra. Those on heart or blood pressure medications should only take ephedra under medical supervision.

Recently, several vitamin companies have introduced products that combine many of the antioxidants with other medicinal herbs. If any are available at your health-food store, you might be able to fulfill the foregoing recommendations with just one type of tablet or capsule.

Proanthocyanidin, a type of bioflavonoid, is an exciting new antioxidant, discovered more than thirty years ago by French professor Jack Masquelier, Ph.D., at the University of Bordeaux. After extensive testing—it is considered to be one of the most investigated nutritional supplements on earth—it is being sold in the United States under the brand name *Pycnogenol,* or as *grape seed extract.* The latter may be more difficult to find in health food stores, but is less expensive, and research has shown it to be even stronger than Pycnogenol. While both are natural plant products in the bioflavonoid "family," Pycnogenol is made from the bark of the European coastal pine tree and its more potent counterpart comes from the seeds of grapes.

Proanthocyanidin is fifty times more powerful an antioxidant than vitamin E and twenty times more than vitamin C. The earliest clinical tests verified its use for improving conditions of the arteries and capillaries, in prevention of infections, as an anti-inflammatory (especially for arthritis), and for anti-aging. Most European physicians consider it to be their first choice for hay fever, and it is also widely used for asthma. Like many other bioflavinoids, this substance is helpful in treating allergies because it prevents the release of histamine. One 100-mg capsule daily would be a good addition to a daily preventive antioxidant regimen. Sinus Survival Grape Seed Extract can be obtained through Klabin Marketing (see "Product Index.")

For readers whose primary complaint is a terrible postnasal drip, or just a lot of clear nasal mucus drainage without a sinus infection, an effective remedy might be *Omega-3 fatty acids* contained in fish oil. They can be found in the store as Super EPA (300 mg) and several other products. Begin with a dosage of two or three capsules a day, then add one a day up to eight or ten capsules or until your symptoms have improved. Then maintain this dosage for at least a month before gradually tapering back down to one capsule a day. If you are a good candidate for the fish oil treatment, you might have several of the following symptoms: dry eyes; dry mouth or excessive thirst; becoming easily cold or easily overheated; dry skin everywhere except face and scalp, which are too oily; cracking on the sides of your heels and fingertips; breaking of fingernails (in layers); rough skin on your thighs, buttocks, and the backs of your arms. The most common side effect of this treatment is belching. This can be minimized by refrigerating the capsules and taking them cold. Diarrhea and a flulike syndrome are also possibilities. Fish oil has also been found to be effective for the treatment of arthritis and chronic urticaria (hives).

Flaxseed oil is another fatty acid whose therapeutic benefits are very similar to those of fish oil. In addition, it can lower cholesterol and promote soft-tissue healing. You cannot cook with it; it must be refrigerated; and the recommended dosage is one tablespoon twice a day.

Other natural remedies for chronic sinusitis and the other respiratory conditions are *peppermint oil, eucalyptus oil,* and *camphorated salve* (Tiger Balm). I put a very small amount (one drop) of peppermint oil on my fingertip, then wipe it around the *outside* of both nostrils. The oil, which acts as a stimulant and decongestant, seems to improve circulation to the nasal and sinus mucous membranes. This enhances the effect of breathing clean and moist air. I like to spray my nose with the saline spray or stand in front of the humidifier and then apply the peppermint oil. It feels wonderful! The Tiger Balm seems to work on the same principle for your lungs. With sinusitis, bronchitis, or asthma I recommend applying it to your chest two or three times a day.

Eucalyptus oil has a similar effect. It can be inhaled either with or without steam, although the former method seems to be most effective. I've recommended putting a few drops in the Steam Inhaler, in the cup provided for this purpose in the Bionaire humidifier, or in a steam room. Without steam, the eucalyptus can simply be applied to a tissue, which you can then hold in front of your nose, while breathing through your nose (if it isn't too congested) for a few minutes. After an initial cough, this usually feels very soothing to the entire respiratory tract, while very effectively relieving nasal congestion, sinus headaches, and the symptoms of asthma and bronchitis. There are approximately 730 different varieties of eucalyptus trees, but only eleven are rated medicinal by the U.S. and British pharmacopeia (drug directory). The eucalyptus oil that I recommend, called V-VAX, is rated number one. I have tried others that are not as effective in treating the respiratory symptoms. V-VAX can also be used as a non-toxic germicide for cuts, burns, and cold sores; and as an effective topical pain reliever for arthritis and muscle soreness. It is available in some health-food stores.

The *Sinus Survival Spray* mentioned briefly in Chapter 5 has been a highly effective recent addition to the Sinus Survival Program. Dr. Steve Morris and I have been using it on ourselves and recommending it to our patients for more than two years, with excellent results. In addition to saline, which makes up the bulk of the spray, the ingredients include:

- goldenseal: acts as an anti-inflammatory;
- selenium: a powerful antioxidant with anti-inflammatory capability;
- aloe vera: has anti-fungal properties and relieves irritation;
- grapefruit seed extract: an excellent anti-fungal.

The first three ingredients are all very healing to the nasal mucous membranes. I've even used this spray as an eye drop and found it extremely soothing for dry and irritated eyes caused by air pollution and arid conditions. When the spray bottle is turned upside down, it can function as an eyedropper. The selenium has allowed the product to be used as part of an allergy treatment program as well as for sinusitis.

The spray will soon be available in some health food stores or through Klabin Marketing.

EXERCISE/PHYSICAL ACTIVITY

"Unhappy people, I am convinced, would increase their happiness more by walking six miles every day, than by any conceivable change in philosophy." So said Bertrand Russell, one of the brilliant minds of our century, who died at the age of ninety-eight. Other benefits of exercise, as compiled by Robert A. Anderson, M.D., are:

I. **Dissipation** of tension; **decreased** sympathetic nervous system activity, fight/flight response, depression, anxiety, smoking, drug use; **increased** self-esteem, positive attitudes, joy, spontaneity, mental acuity, mental function, aerobic capacity, sense of energy; **improved** quality of sleep.

II. **Decreased** back pain; **increased** muscular strength and flexibility; **prevention** of osteoporosis.

III. **Decreased** blood pressure; **increased** oxygen–carrying capacity (oxygen in the bloodstream).

IV. **Decreased** LDL cholesterol (bad cholesterol), triglycerides, glucose, insulin, cortisol; **increased** HDL cholesterol (good cholesterol).

V. **Decreased** recurrence of myocardial infarcts (heart attacks), angina, ischemic heart disease, strokes.

VI. **Decreased** incidence of cancer, free radical populations.

VII. **Decreased** weight; increased lean/fat ratio.

VIII. **Increased** longevity (least fit have a mortality rate 3.5 times that of most fit).

A 1993 study performed on both symptomatic and asymptomatic individuals infected with the HIV virus, by the Departments of Psychiatry, Psychology, and Medicine at the University of Miami School of Medicine, found substantial evidence to conclude that the effects of exercise benefit the psychologic and immunologic status of people suffering from chronic disease.

No discussion of physical health would be complete without including the subject of exercise or physical activity. Yet in spite of the multitude of proven benefits, Americans live in a relatively sedentary society. It is our children, especially, who are getting fatter, weaker, and slower than ever before. The Chrysler Fund's ten-year Amateur Athletic Union Youth Fitness Study found that the number of children and adolescents with "satisfactory" fitness levels dropped from 43 percent in 1980 to 32 percent in 1990. That means two-thirds of the 10 million children tested could not meet minimum standards for strength, flexibility, and endurance. The problem is, as you might have guessed from the foregoing list of exercise benefits, that *unfit means unhealthy*.

We watch an average of more than four hours of television every day, yet the majority of adults cite lack of time as the most frequent reason for not exercising.

Studies have shown that sedentary people, on average, don't live as long or enjoy as good health as those who get regular aerobic exercise: brisk walking, running, swimming, cycling, or similar workouts. Some researchers now believe that getting no exercise might be a more significant risk factor for decreased life expectancy than the *combined* risks of cigarette smoking, high cholesterol, being overweight, and high blood pressure.

The word *aerobic* literally means "with oxygen," and is used to refer to prolonged exercise that requires extra oxygen to supply energy to the muscles through the metabolizing of carbohydrates and fat. In general, aerobic activity causes moderate shortness of breath, perspiring, and the doubling of the resting pulse rate. A few words of conversation should be possible at the height of activity. This is the type of exercise that produces the greatest benefits to the cardiovascular system and provides more oxygen to every other part of the body. The long-term results include slower heart rate, greater cardiac (heart) efficiency, lower blood pressure, and greater physical fitness. If you are looking to decrease the effects of chronic sinusitis (or any other chronic condition) and attain a greater overall feeling of well-being, I recommend a regular program of exercise, preferably aerobic.

This does *not* have to entail a great deal of time. Keep in mind the factors of fun ("What activity would I like to do?" or "What might feel good to me?") and convenience ("How can this be done in the least amount of time?" or "How can I best fit this into my schedule?"). A minimum program of aerobic exercise need consist of only three thirty-minute workouts weekly, maintaining your fitness heart rate two-thirds of that time. To determine this heart rate, use the following formula: 220 minus your age multiplied by 65 to 85 percent equals your fitness heart rate. For example, a 40-year-old's fitness heart rate is between 117 and

153 beats per minute. You have to know how to take your pulse (using your index and middle fingers, feel the pulse either on the thumb side of your wrist or at your neck just below the jaw) and you need a watch with a second hand. Count the number of beats in six seconds and multiply that number by ten to determine your heart rate in beats per minute. When you have attained your fitness heart rate (after about five to ten minutes of exercising), try to maintain it for at least twenty minutes. It is also beneficial to cool down (slower heart rate and less intensity of exercise) for five to ten minutes following the twenty minutes at the fitness rate. Studies have shown that several short daily sessions (three 10-minute exercise sessions separated by at least four hours) can improve exercise performance and weight-loss results. Multiple short sessions of exercise increase aerobic capacity 57 percent, as much as a single long (30-minute) session.

The most convenient forms of aerobic exercise involving the least amount of wear and tear on the body are brisk walking, hiking, swimming, and cycling. If you have easy access to regular cross-country skiing, add that to the list. I no longer recommend running, after seeing too many patients with running-related complaints, usually involving the knees and feet. For year-round cycling, try either a good ten-speed with a turbo trainer for indoor cycling or a stationary bike. Treadmill, rowing, stairclimb, and cross-country ski machines also offer an opportunity for excellent indoor aerobic exercise, as do low-impact aerobics classes. There are several sports played one-on-one or in teams— such as racquetball, handball, badminton, tennis (singles), and basketball—that have the potential for providing a good aerobic workout. Exercise outdoors if you live or work where it is convenient and safe to do so (specifically with regard to automobile traffic and outdoor air quality and temperature). When you exercise, you may increase your intake of air by as much as ten times your level at rest. The combination of fresh air and sunshine provides greater health benefits than indoor exercise. For chronic respiratory disease sufferers, and for those practicing respiratory preventive medicine, air quality is a critical factor in determining where and when to exercise. Ozone, a very harmful air pollutant, is created by the combination of nitrogen oxides, hydrocarbons, and sunlight. A bright sunny day in the downtown area of most large cities would produce high concentrations of ozone. The EPA considers air unhealthy when ozone levels top 0.125 parts per million. However, in a study conducted by New York University's Morton Lippman, M.D., thirty healthy adults showed decreases in lung capacity during a half-hour of exercise at ozone levels below the federal limit.

Writing in the May/June 1989 issue of the journal *Hippocrates,* Benedict Carey suggested scheduling exercise around the rise and fall of pollution levels. In the summer, Carey noted, ozone builds up during the morning, reaches its maximum late in the afternoon, and then ebbs in the evening. In the winter, ozone isn't such a problem, but cold night air can trap a layer of carbon monoxide, nitrogen dioxide, sulfur dioxide, and particulates that can linger into the early morning. A good general practice is to do outdoor exercise in the morning during the summer and in the evening during the winter.

If you are used to walking, biking, or jogging along main roads, lung specialists recommend that you stay away from these high-traffic areas during rush hour. Avoid waiting beside stop signs or stoplights, where carbon monoxide builds up. Henry Going, M.D., a UCLA pulmonologist, says, "I've seen guys jogging in place next to cars at stoplights. You might as well smoke a cigarette." On windy days pollution disperses quickly as you move away from the road. On calm days it can extend about sixty feet from either side of the road.

If all of these concerns pose too great an obstacle, if you live in a highly polluted city, or if you experience a wheeze, cough, or tightness in your chest during your workout, it's time to head indoors for aerobic exercise. Remember that mouth breathing during exercise bypasses the nose and sinuses, your body's natural air filter. Air pollution can therefore more easily aggravate asthma and chronic bronchitis during exercise. Ozone levels in most homes, gyms, and pools are about half that of the outdoors—even less with a good air-conditioning system.

William S. Silvers, M.D., a Denver allergist, has found that many patients with respiratory difficulties who exercise regularly and follow this with a wet steam exposure experience improved breathing, increased mucus flow and expectoration, and had less nasal and throat congestion. He recommends that following your twenty to thirty minutes of aerobic exercise, and after your heart rate has dropped to its pre-exercise level, you have five to ten minutes of exposure to wet steam. This can be done in either a steam room at a health club, the bathroom of your home, with a Steam Inhaler, or by standing over a boiling pot of water with a towel over your head. You should do nasal/chest breathing, which is best performed by taking a deep, slow inhalation through your nose and then breathing out from your chest. Do this as many days as you can, whether you exercise indoors or outdoors.

Moderate exercise is less strenuous than aerobic but still beneficial. In a recent research project at the University of Minnesota School of Public Health, moderate exercise was defined as rapid walking, bowling, gardening, yard work, home repairs, dancing, and home exercise, conducted for about an hour daily. A treadmill test determined that those who got this much leisure-time exercise had healthier hearts than those who got less or none. There was no added benefit in doing more than an hour's worth of physical activity. Robert E. Thayer, Ph.D., a professor of psychology at California State University, Long Beach, has found that brisk walks only ten minutes long can increase people's feelings of energy (sometimes for several hours), reduce tension, and make personal problems appear less serious. Not only does it nourish mind and body, *walking is also by far the easiest, safest, and least expensive (you need only comfortable shoes) form of exercise.* Briskly walking two miles at 3.5 to 4 miles per hour (15-minute miles) burns nearly as many calories as running at a moderate pace, and confers similar fitness benefits. By swinging your arms, you'll burn 5 to 10 percent more calories and get an upper-body workout as well.

Aerobic exercise should precede meals or follow by at least two and a half hours. *Don't begin an aerobic activity in the heat of an emotional crisis, especially if you're very angry.* Wait at least 15 to 20 minutes.

For strengthening and toning, I recommend both push-ups and sit-ups. Remember that with sit-ups you need not raise your trunk any higher than 45 degrees from the floor.

Maintaining and increasing flexibility is an essential part of your overall physical fitness program. Flexibility is the ability to use muscles and joints through their full range of movement. Research has suggested that good muscle elasticity lends agility, a potential for greater speed, and a reduced chance of injury to muscles, tendons, and ligaments. A regular routine of gentle stretching or yoga can be a relaxing and invigorating way to start your day. The books *Stretching* by Bob Anderson, and *Yoga: The Iyengar Way* by Mira, Silva, and Shyam Mehta, are both excellent guides.

Aerobic exercise was an integral part of the program I used to cure my own chronic sinusitis, and it is still a big part of my routine. Initially it requires discipline. Start gradually and try not to push yourself too hard. Exercise does not have to hurt to be beneficial, in spite of the prevalent belief in "no pain, no gain." It won't take long before you start looking forward to it as one of the highlights of your day. The benefits that you will soon realize will help to increase your motivation to continue. You might eventually make it a daily routine, although research has shown no increased cardiovascular benefits beyond five days a week (three times a week is minimum). However, exercise does much more than merely benefit your heart. As these aerobic workouts strengthen your heart and lungs directly, your ability to provide oxygen to every part of your body is enhanced—and this, after all, is the scientific basis of physical health. As a human animal, you can experience many of life's greatest pleasures only through your body. Regular exercise can add immeasurably to your enjoyment of life and heighten your sense of well-being.

SLEEP/REST

Perhaps the most overlooked and powerful means of strengthening your immune system is sleep. The average person requires between eight and nine hours of uninterrupted sleep, yet in our sleep-deprived nation, we average between six and eight hours. And there are an estimated 50 million Americans who would be pleased to sleep even that many hours. They suffer from insomnia, defined by Neil B. Kavey, M.D., director of the Sleep Disorders Center at Columbia-Presbyterian Hospital in New York City, as the inability to sleep at night, resulting in fatigue the next day.

Lack of sleep is almost always a factor in causing colds and sinus infections, and getting additional sleep is correspondingly an essential component of the treatment. While it obviously lowers immunity, sleep deprivation can also cause a decrease in productivity, creativity, and job performance. In the majority of cases, insomnia is related to a specific event or situation that induces stress. While stress-induced insomnia is often transient, it may persist well beyond the event that precipitated the condition and become a chronic problem. Overstimulation of the nervous system (produced by caffeine, salt, sugar), or simply the fear that you can't fall asleep, are other common causes.

Although researchers are still not exactly sure why sleep is necessary and how much we need, they have identified two types of sleep: heavy and light. During heavier sleep, called NonRapid Eye Movement Sleep (NREM), your body's self-repair healing mechanisms get revitalized, enabling your body to repair itself. During lighter, Rapid Eye Movement Sleep (REM), you dream more and release stress and tension.

Sleeping pills have been the conventional medical treatment for insomnia, but as with almost all medications, there are unpleasant side effects to contend with, not to mention the dependence they can create with this condition.

A more natural approach begins with a regular bedtime every

night, as you begin to attune yourself to nature's rhythms. According to the teachings of Ayurvedic medicine, the traditional medicine of India, the circadian rhythm, caused by the earth rotating on its axis every twenty-four hours, has a counterpart in the human body. Modern science has shown that many neurological and endocrine functions follow this twenty-four-hour circadian rhythm, including the sleep-wakefulness cycle. Ayurveda teaches that the ideal bedtime for the deepest sleep and for being in sync with this natural rhythm is 10 P.M. Unfortunately, most people with insomnia dread bedtime and end up going to bed between 10 P.M. and 2 A.M., when sleep tends to be somewhat lighter and more active. According to Ayur-Veda, eight hours of sleep starting at 9:30 P.M. is twice as restful as eight hours beginning at 2 A.M. It is also important in resetting your biological clock to get up early and at the same time every day, regardless of when you go to bed. Establishing an early wake-up time (6 or 7 A.M.) is essential for overcoming insomnia. You'll eventually begin to feel sleepy earlier in the evening. Even if you are not actually sleeping by 10 P.M., you'll benefit just by resting in bed at that hour.

Other natural remedies include:

- vitamin B complex, 50mg 2x/day;
- calcium, 800–1,000mg a day; (a deficiency of either or both of the above is associated with insomnia);
- chamomile, passionflower, hops, skullcap, and valerian herbs; they are natural sedatives that do not alter the quality of sleep the way prescription and over-the-counter drugs do; they can all be taken as a tea, while valerian and passionflower are available in stronger dosages in a tincture form;
- hot bath or hot tub;
- breathing exercises and/or meditation to relax muscles and relieve tension.

Most important, don't worry about lost sleep. Anxiety is, in most cases, what caused the problem in the first place. If you can learn to relax without drugs, you will have cured your insomnia, and at the same time, given your immune system a powerful boost. The following chapters can help you to achieve this goal.

However, before shifting your focus from the body to the mind, there still may be symptoms to treat. In fact, some of them may be partially responsible for your insomnia, and for making you feel miserable during the day as well. Besides the recommendations that have already been presented in this chapter, the following sections on allergies, asthma, bronchitis, and colds offer you additional natural options for obtaining even greater relief from each of these uncomfortable conditions.

ALLERGY TREATMENT

In Chapter 5 I outlined the conventional medical treatment for allergies, hay fever, and allergic rhinitis. If you are interested in a complement to that regimen or in a non-medicated alternative, it is possible to treat allergies effectively without drugs. So far in this chapter, the dietary, antioxidant (vitamins C, A [beta-carotene], E, selenium, and zinc), and water recommendations, as well as the avoidance of certain foods—milk, corn, eggs, and wheat especially—are all helpful in treating allergies.

An air cleaner or a negative-ion generator can also have a significant impact. Dr. ShihWen Huang, a professor at the Shands Teaching Hospital at the University of Florida in Gainesville, conducted an independent study on ninety children afflicted with perennial allergic rhinitis (forty-three of them also had asthma) and their families, for at least three years. He placed an air cleaner, without ionization, in their homes for a full year. Their allergic symptoms were scored weekly by the parents, and the patients were evaluated every three months. The results of the symptom score showed: (1) improvement in quality of sleep (less snoring or mouth breathing) in 98 percent of the children; (2) improvement of allergic symptoms: sneezing 80 percent, scratchy throat 75 percent, nasal congestion 70 percent, cough 75 percent, wheezing 70 percent, better behavior or mood 65 percent, sinus infection 50 percent, postnasal drip 40 percent. The overall improvement was most apparent in 85 percent of the children during the first four months of the study. The parents also reported as a group: (1) 72 percent reduction in work days lost; (2) 43 percent decrease in school days missed; (3) 49 percent reduction in emergency room visits; (4) 63 percent decrease in clinic visits related to allergy problems; (5) 12 percent increase in clinic visits for non-allergy-related problems; (6) 76 percent reduction in over-the-counter drugs purchased; (7) 43 percent reduction in prescription drugs purchased. Dr. Huang's conclusions: (1) significant beneficial effects of adding an air-cleaner unit in the bedroom of allergic children with perennial rhinitis were observed with proper monitoring; (2) more frequent change of the filter (every four months) may maximize the effect of air cleaner due to the difference in indoor pollution in each household.

Although I know of no similar study using negative-ion generators as air cleaners, I would strongly suspect that the benefits would be even more impressive.

Modified cleansing diets are also helpful during your high allergy seasons. These should be administered by a nutritionally oriented physician or a naturopath.

Ruling out food allergy is another suggestion. Food allergies are often to foods that you crave. Many people with pollen allergy are also allergic to foods, particulary dairy and wheat. Doris Rapp, author of *Allergies and Your Family,* describes a fast method of spotting allergy culprits in foods. She says, "Before you have eaten anything, take your pulse in the morning and count the number of heartbeats for a full minute. Next, eat the food you wish to test on an empty stomach. Wait fifteen to thirty minutes and then take your pulse again. If it has gone up fifteen to twenty beats per minute, chances are you ate something to which you are sensitive."

Some people might even be allergic to water, and it can cause reactions similar to food allergies. Tap water, with its many chemicals, is causing problems for a growing number of people. If you suspect food allergy but are unable to determine the cause, you might consult with a clinical ecologist. These physicians have a more comprehensive perspective than conventional allergists, along with greater recognition of environmental allergens. To learn more about clinical ecologists or to find one in your area, write to: The American Academy of Environmental Medicine, P.O. Box 16106, Denver, CO 80216.

Other than a weakened immune system, physiologic factors that have been found to contribute to allergies are a diminished secretion of hydrochloric acid in the stomach and a magnesium deficiency, or a magnesium/calcium imbalance. In addition to the vitamins and minerals that have already been mentioned, I recommend the following when treating allergies:

- vitamin B-6, 200mg 2x/day (bolsters immune system);
- pantothenic acid, 500mg 3x/day following meals (strengthens adrenal glands);
- a combination of quercetin (a bioflavonoid usually found in blue-green algae) and bromelain, total daily dosage between 1,000 and 2,000mg divided into three to six doses (a natural antihistamine);
- freeze-dried nettles, 300mg 1–3x/day (a natural antihistamine);
- hydrochloric acid tablets, 1 or 2 before meals (stimulates digestion);
- licorice *(Glycyrrhiza glabra),* 10 to 20 drops 3x/day (reduces inflammation of mucous membranes; don't use if you have high blood pressure or an enlarged prostate);
- magnesium citrate or aspartate, 400mg 1–3x/day (natural antihistamine);
- proanthocyanidin, 100mg 3x/day.

There are also a number of products containing ephedra in combination with other herbs, such as Decongest Herbal and

Allerex, that I would suggest taking if you are very congested. In Chapter 14, I present several other options for physically treating allergies with osteopathic techniques, Chinese medicine, reflexology, and homeopathic remedies. These can all be done in conjunction with the regimen presented in this section. I know this seems like a lot of pills to take, and it is, but it's also guaranteed to reduce your allergy symptoms significantly without any unpleasant side effects.

Although I'm not personally familiar with anyone who has tried it, I was intrigued by the following remedy for allergies found in *Prevention* magazine: Find a fresh horseradish root and cut a slice out of the middle about the size of a thick potato chip; chop it up very fine. Put it in a blender with about 2 or 3 tablespoons of apple cider vinegar. Blend for about 30 seconds. Next, take a full tablespoon of the mixture, put it in your mouth, and hold it there for about 2 minutes, and then swallow it. Not the greatest taste, but the author claims fantastic results. He followed this procedure for two consecutive mornings and one evening and was totally cured of his allergies for five years, at which time he took a "booster" and is still fine four years later.

In the following chapters you will learn how to use your mind and spirit together with this physical approach to cure allergies. It may not be as simple as the horseradish remedy, but your level of growth and healing will be far greater.

ASTHMA

In the midst of an acute asthma attack, there is no better treatment than the lifesaving medications of conventional medicine. Many asthmatics have experienced the terrifying feeling of not being able to breathe and have visited the local emergency room more than once. The treatment plan that I am proposing can help to prevent these crises from occurring. If you practice the entire holistic regimen as outlined in Part II of this book, eventually you should be able to gradually stop using long-term medications and inhalers, some of which may be prolonging or even aggravating your asthma (particularly chronic use of beta-agonist sprays—see Chapter 5). I recommend that you find a physician who is willing to work with you on implementing this approach. The majority of doctors who treat asthma have a high level of frustration in dealing with this problem (although not as high as yours), and might be open to trying a new approach. If you are unable to find such a physician, contact the American Academy of Environmental Medicine or the American Holistic Medical Association (see Chapter 15).

As you start the program, maintain your present medications, but within a short time you can begin to very gradually taper off. The holistic approach is directed at mitigating and eliminating as many of the causes of asthma as you can identify. Since air pollution is a primary reason for the present asthma epidemic, I suggest a *negative-ion generator* in your bedroom and workplace. Refer to Chapter 7 and do a thorough job of creating a *healthy home,* as well as learn to become more aware of air conditions, both indoor and outdoor. Pay particular attention to air quality before exercising outdoors.

Moisture and steam are quite helpful in healing the scarred and inflamed mucous membrane lining the bronchial tubes. Negative ions, antioxidants, and nutritional supplements can also contribute to healing. As I have mentioned earlier in this chapter, many of the vitamins, minerals, and herbs can also help to strengthen your immune system. Together with a healthy *diet* (medicinal foods that can benefit asthmatics include cayenne, garlic, and ginger), adequate *water* intake, a good *exercise* program, and the *elimination of foods* that might be triggering an allergic reaction (dairy, wheat, and soy), you'll be off to a great start.

On the cellular level, biopsies performed on the lungs of asthmatics have revealed vitamin and mineral deficiencies, especially magnesium. *Magnesium,* which has both an antihistamine and a mild bronchodilation effect, has been used very successfully in the treatment of asthma since the 1930s. Virtually all of the currently used asthma drugs draw magnesium out of the cells lining the airway, creating a deficiency that in turn causes bronchial constriction. Magnesium given concurrently with the drugs can enhance their action while minimizing toxicity. But most important, magnesium can be used preventively in treating asthma.

Omega-3 fatty acids, found in fish oil (the same ingredient contained in Super EPA, p. 151), act as natural anti-inflammatories and can be quite beneficial in treating asthma. Fish oils can moderate the late-phase reaction of asthma. (Asthma attacks often include an acute inflammatory response and a secondary, late-phase reaction, which can occur up to twenty-four hours later and last for weeks.) These fatty acids are found in dark-meat fishes such as salmon and tuna. If you regularly eat these fish, take 6 grams of fish oil a day, and up to 12 grams a day for non–fish eaters. Comparable amounts of Omega-3 fatty acids can be obtained from 3 tablespoons of *flaxseed oil* a day. Asthmatics who are sensitive to aspirin should not take Omega-3 oils since they may intensify this problem.

A relatively new treatment involves *platelet-activating-factor (PAF) inhibitors*. Platelets are blood cells important to wound healing and blood clotting. But they also stimulate inflammation and trigger allergies. Alan Gaby, M.D., current president of the American Holistic Medical Association, author of *Preventing and Reversing Osteoporosis,* and one of the world's foremost authorities on nutritional medicine, believes that PAFs play a major role in causing almost all food allergies. When PAF levels are lowered, allergy and asthma symptoms can be eased. The Chinese herb gingko biloba and the shark oil extract Ecomer are both effective PAF inhibitors.

In addition to the *antioxidant* vitamins C, beta carotene, and E (vitamin E neutralizes the damaging effects of ozone), minerals (zinc and selenium), and *proanthocyanidin* in the dosages previously mentioned, I suggest the following:

- magnesium citrate, aspartate, or chelate, 500mg 2–3×/day;
- vitamin B-6, 50mg 2×/day;

- vitamin B-12, 500mcg taken sublingually (under tongue);
- ginkgo biloba, 40mg of 24 percent standardized extract 3×/day (a Chinese herb);
- Coleus forskholi, 3–4mg/day (an Ayurvedic herb);
- N-Acetylcysteine (NAC), 500mg 2×/day (an amino acid, a good mucolytic);
- Ecomer, 50mg 3×/day (a shark oil extract).

The first five substances on this list are contained in one product called Ventimax, made by CMC. It is available in many health food stores.

Products containing the herb ephedra or Ma huang can also help in treating asthma, although they should not be taken if you have high blood pressure. The peak bronchodilation effect from ephedra occurs in one hour and lasts for about five hours. The ephedra dose should have an ephedrine content of 12.5 to 25mg and be taken 2 to 3×/day.

Emotional stress is a major factor in both causing and exacerbating asthma. Studies have shown that asthmatics who do daily yoga training can significantly increase their lung function and their exercise capacity. Yoga not only improves the way a person breathes, it is also a highly effective relaxation technique. It will be discussed along with other methods of stress reduction in the following chapters.

If you adhere closely to only that part of the holistic treatment for asthma described in this chapter, you will have a reasonable chance of being free of daily use of asthma medications within three months. You will want to have them available, however, because it can take approximately nine months to one year for the bronchial mucous membranes to heal completely. Until then you will still be at greater risk for experiencing an asthma attack. In the meantime, you can reduce that risk much further if you commit to working on the emotional origins of your asthma as diligently as you have to the physical and environmental.

BRONCHITIS

The physical and environmental aspects of the holistic medical treatment for both acute and chronic bronchitis do not differ substantially from the regimen prescribed for sinusitis and asthma. Acute bonchitis is very similar to acute sinusitis, except that the infection is focused in the lungs. In a majority of cases, I believe that the infection actually exists simultaneously in both the sinuses and lungs. The treatment for acute bronchitis should therefore include all of the medicinal herbs (garlic, echinacea, goldenseal), vitamins, minerals, and antioxidants that I have recommended for acute sinusitis. I also make the same suggestion regarding antibiotics as I have for sinus infections. If you have acute bronchitis (or take an antibiotic for another reason) once or twice a year, then it's fine to treat your infection with an antibiotic along with the natural regimen. Remember to take acidophilus along with the drug. Moisture and steam are just as helpful for bronchitis as they are for a sinus infection.

Since chronic bronchitis combines elements of both chronic sinusitis and asthma, I recommend a synthesis of both of these treatment plans in healing this challenging condition. It involves taking lots of pills (see chart on p. 175), but for someone who suffers from the debilitating effects of chronic bronchitis, it should definitely be worth it. Before doing anything else, you must completely *stop smoking*. Negative ions, steam, a nutritious diet, adequate water, and a moderate exercise program are all essential. But perhaps the most valuable aspects of the treatment program for chronic bronchitis are *postural drainage* (described with diagrams in Chapter 5), a natural method of "irrigating" or emptying the lungs of tenacious mucus, and the *amino acid N-Acetylcysteine (NAC)*. This substance has been clinically useful throughout the world as an agent to reduce the mucous viscosity in lung disorders. (I included it in the treatment of asthma.) NAC also has an impressive ability to chelate (absorb) heavy metals and to deactivate environmental carcinogenic chemicals. It acts as a potent antioxidant and anti-inflammatory, and in so doing can help to prevent infectious recurrences, diminished lung function, scarring of lung tissue, and lung cancer. The dosage for NAC is 500mg 3×/day.

If you have a resistant case of chronic bronchitis and are in the position to do so, I would recommend moving to an area with optimum healthy air. Ultimately that may be a more valuable therapeutic measure than any of the other physical and environmental components of the holistic program for treating any of the chronic respiratory diseases. Your greatest challenge will then be to find that "perfect" place.

COLDS

The common cold is usually the trigger for causing acute sinusitis, acute bronchitis, and an asthma attack. Since these conditions often lead to chronic sinusitis, chronic bronchitis, and chronic asthma, it is extremely helpful to be able to either prevent colds or greatly reduce their adverse effects. Colds almost always result from an *overload of stress—physical, emotional, or both:* eating poorly, not enough sleep, heavy exposure to cold viruses and polluted air, too much exercise, and most often, too much work or overextending yourself. In my own experience and that of my patients, attempting to do too many things at once is the weight that consistently tips the scale and weakens the immune system just enough to bring on a cold. Early recognition of the factors responsible for colds will allow you to make choices that can prevent the infection from ever getting a strong foothold in your body and making you sick. The remainder of Part II will teach you to heighten your emotional awareness to a point where you can recognize the emotional triggers of a cold early enough to defuse or release them. For nearly five years after curing my chronic sinusitis, I did not have one cold! This was a major contributor to my being able to maintain healthy sinuses.

However, it takes time and practice to finely tune your emotional "antennae." If you're not quite there yet, the first physical symptoms of a cold are usually a sore throat, fatigue, and feeling weak or achy. If you respond quickly enough to the earliest signs of a cold, you can usually avoid the full force of the infection and not infrequently prevent the cold in its entirety. At that first hint of a sore throat or generalized achiness, I suggest the following:

* rest and get more sleep;
* vitamin C, between 15 and 20,000mg in the first twenty-four hours; can be taken either 5,000mg 3 or 4×/day, 2,000mg every 2 hours, or 1,000mg every waking hour; very gradually taper this dose over the next 3 to 5 days;
* Yin Chiao, a Chinese herb, 3 to 5 bottles/day in the first forty-eight hours (each bottle has 8 tablets);
* garlic, eaten raw or in liquid or capsule;
* echinacea, 1 dropperful 3×/day for 3 to 5 days;
* goldenseal, 1 dropperful 3×/day for 3 to 5 days;
* beta carotene, vitamin E, selenium, and zinc, in same dosages as for acute sinusitis;
* gargle with salt water, use saline nasal spray, and Sucrets or throat lozenges;
* lots of warm or hot liquids; "Traditional Medicinal" teas; gingerroot or peppermint tea, can also include ginger, honey, lemon, cayenne, cinnamon, and a teaspoon of brandy;
* a hot bath and steam;
* the "homeopathic vitamin Cs," Aconitum (monkshood) and Ferrum phos (iron phosphate); or the homeopathic oscillococcinum;
* diet: eliminate dairy products and eat lighter foods, less protein.

The sooner you act, the more effectively you will be able to prevent the cold. Keep in mind the basic objective of the physical aspect of holistic medical treatment—*love your body*. By creating the uncomfortable symptoms of a cold, your body is sending you a very strong message. There is a need for nurturing that isn't being met. You've been "doing" too much and not caring enough for yourself. Your actions and behavior, in conjunction with your genetic and emotional makeup, have combined to create an imbalance that manifests as physical discomfort. If balance is not restored and the body's warnings are not heeded, the problem can progress into a dis-ease (such as chronic sinusitis)—a persistent state of imbalance and physical disharmony.

Your body has an innate intelligence and is perfectly capable of healing itself. It knows precisely what is required in order to heal, and it will communicate those needs to you on a regular basis. It will tell you if the air you're breathing or the food you're eating doesn't agree with you. But in order for you to hear the messages, you must learn to become better attuned to your body and learn its language. You will have to make a greater commitment to nurturing yourself. When you do, you will experience a degree of physical well-being you haven't felt in years. From this new state of "normal" you will become much more sensitive to any imbalance in your body. For those of you with a chronic respiratory disease, or any other "incurable" condition, you have to become better listeners and better nurturers before you can cure your ailment. In the process of learning healthy behavior and how to better respond to your body's needs, you will gradually become a much higher priority in your life and your dis-ease will disappear.

Before reading any further, I would suggest implementing the recommendations in this chapter. Start slowly and record your progress on the Symptom Chart (pp. 129–30). After three or four weeks you will almost certainly be feeling better. That would be a good time to move on to "Mental Health" and Chapter 10. If you've closely adhered to the program outlined in this chapter (Chapter 8) and there has been very little change, go to Chapter 9 and see if you qualify as a candidate for the candida regimen. Some of you may already suspect you have candidiasis. In that case combine chapters 8 and 9 and follow them concurrently.

Table 8-3

Natural Quick-Fix Symptom Treatment

Cough
gargle, then drink lemon juice and honey (1:1) with a tablespoon of vodka
licorice-based tea
ginger tea
wild cherry bark syrup
Bronchial drops (a homeopathic)
Sinus Survival Cough Syrup and Cough Drops

Fatigue
ginseng
antioxidants, especially vitamin C
folic acid
vitamin B-12 500mcg 2×/day
vitamin B-6 75 to 100mg/day
pantothenic acid 500mg 1 or 2×/day
meditation
exercise
sleep
pace yourself between activity and rest
rule out anemia

Headache
adequate water intake
negative ions
steam
eucalyptus oil
acupressure/reflexology points
hydrotherapy—alternate hot and cold shower
garlic or horseradish (chew it)
calcium/magnesium
quercetin 2 caps 3×/day
Fenu/Thyme (Nature's Way) 2 caps 3×/day
Ginkgo biloba 40mg 3×/day
Feverfew avena 20 drops 3×/day

Runny Nose
adequate water intake

saline spray
ephedra (not with high blood pressure)
nettles 1 cap 3×/day
quercetin 2 tabs 3×/day
vitamin C 6,000 to 10,000mg/day

Sneezing
adequate water intake
acupressure/reflexology points
nettles 2 caps 2 to 3×/day
quercetin + bromelain 2 caps 2 to 3×/day before meals

Sore Throat
gargle with lemon juice and honey (1:1)
gargle with pinch of cayenne + 1 tsp. salt in 8oz. water
licorice-based tea (Long Life, Traditional Medicinals, or Throat Coat)
lozenges (Zand Eucalyptus, Holistic brand Propolis)
zinc picolinate 30mg 3×/day
garlic 2 caps 3×/day
Zand Throat Spray

Stuffy Nose
adequate water intake
hot tea with lemon
hot chicken soup
steam
hydrotherapy (hot water from shower) or hot compresses
eucalyptus oil
horseradish
acupressure/reflexology points
massage
orgasm
exercise
garlic
onions
cayenne pepper
Breathe Right™—External Nasal Dilator
no ice-cold drinks
no dairy
no gluten: wheat, rye, oats, barley
ephedra 20 to 30 drops 4×/day for 2 to 3 days (max.)
rule out allergies

papaya enzyme tablets 1 or 2 4×/day (dissolved in mouth)—use also for ear congestion, sinus congestion, and sinus pain

anger release, especially punching

Wheezing

ephedra 12.5 to 25mg 2 or 3×/day (can increase heart rate and anxiety —don't use with high blood pressure)

lobelia 25 drops in mint tea every $^1/_2$ to 1 hr. (may cause nausea)

no glutens or sulfites

no milk or dairy

caffeine

magnesium glycinate, citrate, or aspartate 250mg every 3 hrs.

vitamin B-6 200mg 2×/day

vitamin B-12 500mcg (sublingual) 2×/day

vitamin C 3,000 to 5,000 3×/day

selenium 200mcg 1×/day

onions

The Physical and Environmental Health Components of the *Sinus Survival Program* for Treating and Preventing *Sinusitis, Bronchitis,* and *Colds*

	PREVENTIVE MAINTENANCE	TREATING AN INFECTION
Sleep	7–9 hrs/day; No alarm clock	8–10+ hrs/day
Negative ions or air cleaner	Continuous operation; use ions especially with air conditioning	continuous operation
Humidifier, warm mist	Use during dry conditions, especially in winter if heat is on and in summer if air conditioner is on	Continuous operation
Saline nasal spray (SS spray)	Use daily, especially with dirty and/or dry air	Use daily, every 2–3 hours
Steam	Use as needed with dirty and/or dry air	Use daily, 2–4 x/day
Nasal Irrigation	Use as needed with dirty and/or dry air	Use daily, 2–4 x/day after steam
Water, bottled or filtered	Drink $^1/_2$ oz./lb. body weight; with exercise, drink $^2/_3$ oz./lb.	$^1/_2$ to $^2/_3$ oz./lb. body weight
Diet	↑ Fresh fruit, vegetables, whole grains, fiber ↓ sugar, dairy, caffeine, alcohol	No sugar, dairy
Exercise, preferably aerobic	Minimum 20–30 min., 3–5 x/week; avoid outdoors if high pollution	No aerobic; moderate walking only
✳7 Postural Drainage		

	ADULTS		CHILDREN (Over 3 yrs. of Age)		PREGNANCY	
	① PREVENTIVE MAINTENANCE	FOR SINUSITIS, BRONCHITIS, OR A COLD	PREVENTION	FOR SINUSITIS, BRONCHITIS, OR A COLD	PREVENTION	FOR SINUSITIS, BRONCHITIS, OR A COLD
Vitamin C (polyascorbate or Ester C)	1,000 to 2,000 mg 3x/d	4,000 to 6,000 mg 3x/d	100 to 250 mg 3x/d	500 to 1,000 mg 3x/d	1,000 mg. 2x/d	1,000 mg. 4x/day
Beta Carotene	25,000 I.U. 1 or 2x/d	⊛⑧ 50,000 I.U. 2x/d	5,000 I.U. 1 or 2x/d	10,000 I.U. 2x/d	25,000 I.U. 1x/d	25,000 I.U. 2x/d
Vitamin E	400 I.U. 1 or 2x/d	400 I.U. 2x/d	50 I.U. 1 or 2x/d	200 I.U. 2x/d	200 I.U. 1x/d	200 I.U. 2x/d
Proanthocyanidin (grape seed extract or Pycnogenol)	100 mg 1 or 2x/d	100 mg 3x/d	—	100 mg 1x/d	—	100 mg 1x/d
⊛② Multivitamin	1 to 3x/d	1 to 3x/d	Pediatric Multivitamin		Prenatal Multivitamin with 800 mg Folic acid	
Selenium	100 to 200 mcg/d	200 mcg/d	—	100 mcg/d	25 mcg/d	100 mcg 2x/d
Zinc picolinate	20 to 40 mg/d	40 to 60 mg/d	10 mg/d	10 mg 2x/d	25 mg/d	40 mg/d
Magnesium citrate or aspartate	500 mg/d	500 mg/d	150 to 250 mg/d	300 mg/d	500 mg/d	500 mg/d
Calcium (citrate or hydroxyapatite)	1,000 mg/d; menopause: 1,500 mg/d	1,000 mg/d; menopause: 1,500 mg/d	600 to 800 mg/d from diet		1,200 mg/d	1,200 mg/d

	ADULTS		CHILDREN (Over 3 yrs. of Age)		PREGNANCY	
	PREVENTIVE MAINTENANCE	FOR SINUSITIS, BRONCHITIS, OR A COLD	PREVENTION	FOR SINUSITIS, BRONCHITIS, OR A COLD	PREVENTION	FOR SINUSITIS, BRONCHITIS, OR A COLD
Chromium picolinate	200 mcg/d	200 mcg/d	—	—	in Prenatal Multivitamin	
Garlic	—	1,200 to 2,000 mg 3x/d	—	1,000 mg 3x/d	—	1,200 mg 3x/d
Echinacea	—	200 mg 3x/d or 25 drops 4–5 x/d	—	100 mg 3x/d or 7–10 drops 3x/d	—	200 mg 3x/d or 25 drops 4x/d
✪9 Goldenseal	—	200 mg 3x/d or 20 drops 4–5 x/d	—	100 mg 3x/d or 7–10 drops 3x/d	—	—
Bee propolis	—	500 mg 3x/d	—	200 mg 3x/d or 500 mg 1x/d	—	500 mg 3x/d
Grapefruit (citrus) seed extract	—	100 mg 3x/d or 10 drops in water 3x/d	—	4 drops in water 2x/d	—	100 mg 3x/d or 10 drops in water 3x/d
Flaxseed oil (or Omega-3 fatty acids in fish oil)	2 Tblsp/d	2 Tblsp/d	1 Tblsp/d	1 Tblsp/d	2 Tblsp/d	2 Tblsp/d
✪3 N-acetylcysteine (NAC)	500 mg 3x/d	500 mg 3x/d	—	200 mg 3x/d	—	500 mg 3x/d

	ADULTS		CHILDREN (Over 3 yrs. of Age)		PREGNANCY	
	①PREVENTIVE MAINTENANCE	FOR SINUSITIS, BRONCHITIS, OR A COLD	PREVENTION	FOR SINUSITIS, BRONCHITIS, OR A COLD	PREVENTION	FOR SINUSITIS, BRONCHITIS, OR A COLD
★4 Yin Chiao (1 bottle = 8 tablets)	—	1 bottle 3 to 5x/d for 2 days	—	¹/₂ bottle (4 tablets) 3x/d for 2 days	—	—
★5 Acidophilus (lactobacillus acidophilus and bifidus)	★10 ¹/₂ tsp. in ¹/₂ cup water 2x/d (AM & PM)	¹/₂ tsp. 3x/d or 2 caps 3x/d	★10 ¹/₄ tsp. 2x/d	¹/₄ tsp. 3x/d	★10 ¹/₂ tsp. 2x/d	¹/₂ tsp. 3x/d
★6 Antibiotics						

★1 Use the higher dosages on days of higher stress, less sleep, and increased air pollution
★2 Dosage depends on brand
★3 Use only for preventing and treating chronic bronchitis
★4 Use only at <u>onset</u> of a cold and influenza
★5 Use as part of the treatment program only if candidiasis is suspected
★6 Antibiotics—an option for sinusitis and bronchitis if taken infrequently, i.e., 1 or 2x/ year
★7 Postural drainage for chronic bronchitis only
★8 Use this dosage for maximum of 1 month
★9 Use with caution if you have ragweed allergy
★10 Take this preventive acidophilus for only 2 weeks, 3x/year and when you're taking an antibiotic; refer to p. 215 for more information about acidophilus

The Physical and Environmental Health Components of the *Sinus Survival Program* for Treating and Preventing *Allergies* and *Asthma*

	PREVENTIVE MAINTENANCE	TREATING ALLERGIES & ASTHMA
Sleep	7–9 hrs/day; No alarm clock	8–10+ hrs/day
Negative ions or air cleaner	Continuous operation (use neg. ions, esp. if air conditioner is in use)	continuous operation (esp. during allergy season)
Humidifier, warm mist	Use during dry conditions—in winter if heat is on; in summer if air conditioner is on	
Saline nasal spray (SS spray)	Use daily, several times/day, especially with dirty and/or dry air	
Steam	Use as needed with dirty and/ or dry air	Use daily, 2–4 x/day
Nasal Irrigation (allergies only)	Use as needed with dirty and/ or dry air	Use daily, 2–4 x/day, after steam
Water, bottled or filtered	Drink 1/2 oz./lb. of body weight; with exercise 2/3 oz./lb.	
Diet	Increase fresh fruit, vegetables, whole grains, fiber; cayenne, ginger and garlic for asthma; decrease sugar, dairy, wheat, and alcohol; do food elimination diet to determine any food allergy	
Exercise, prefera- bly aerobic	Minimum 20–30 min., 3–5 x/ week. Avoid outdoors if high pollution and/or pollen	No aerobic; moderate walking OK. Avoid out- doors if high pollution and/or pollen

	ADULTS		CHILDREN (Over 3 yrs. of Age)		PREGNANCY	
	PREVENTIVE MAINTENANCE	TREATING ALLERGIES & ASTHMA	PREVENTION	TREATING ALLERGIES & ASTHMA	PREVENTION	TREATING ALLERGIES & ASTHMA
Vitamin C (polyas-corbate or Ester C)	1,000–2,000 mg 3x/d	3,000–5,000 mg 3x/d	100–250 mg 3x/d	500–1,000 mg 3x/d	1,000 mg. 2x/d	1,000 mg. 4x/day
Beta Carotene	25,000 I.U. 1 or 2x/d	25,000 I.U. 3x/d	5,000 I.U. 1 or 2x/d	10,000 I.U. 2x/d	25,000 I.U. 1x/d	25,000 I.U. 2x/d
Vitamin E	400 I.U. 1 or 2x/d	400 I.U. 2x/d	50 I.U. 1 or 2x/d	200 I.U. 2x/d	200 I.U. 1x/d	200 I.U. 2x/d
Proanthocy-anidin (grape seed extract or Pycnoge-nol)	100 mg 1 or 2x/d	100 mg 3x/d	—	100 mg 1x/d	—	100 mg 1x/d
Multi-vitamin	1–3x/d	1–3x/d	Pediatric Multi-vitamin		Prenatal Multi-vitamin with 800 mg Folic acid	
Selenium	100–200 mcg/d	200 mcg/d	—	100 mcg/d	25 mcg/d	100 mcg 2x/d
Zinc picolinate	20–40 mg/d	40–60 mg/d	10 mg/d	10 mg 2x/d	25 mg/d	40 mg/d
Magnesium citrate or aspartate	500 mg/d	500 mg 2 or 3x/d	150 to 250 mg/d	300 mg/d	500 mg/d	500 mg/d
Calcium (citrate or hydroxy-apatite)	1,000 mg/d; meno-pause: 1,500 mg/d	1,000 mg/d; meno-pause: 1,500 mg/d	600–800 mg/d from diet		1,200 mg/d	1,200 mg/d
Chromium picolinate	200 mcg/d	200 mcg/d	—	—	in Prenatal Multi-vitamin	

	ADULTS		CHILDREN (Over 3 yrs. of Age)		PREGNANCY	
	★① PREVENTIVE MAINTENANCE	TREATING ALLERGIES & ASTHMA	PREVENTION	TREATING ALLERGIES & ASTHMA	PREVENTION	TREATING ALLERGIES & ASTHMA
Vitamin B-6	50 mg 2x/d	200 mg 2x/d	10 mg 1x/d	25 mg 1x/d	25 mg 1x/d	25 mg 2x/d
Garlic	—	1,2000 to 2,000 mg 3x/d	—	1,000 mg 3x/d	—	1,200 mg 3x/d
★② Ephedra or Ma huang	—	12.5 to 25 mg 2 or 3x/d	—	5 mg 2x/d	—	—
★③ Licorice (Glycyrrhiza glabra)	—	★⑦ 10 to 20 drops 3x/d	—	5–10 drops 2 to 3x/d	—	—
Nettles, freeze dried	—	300 mg 1 to 3x/d	—	—	—	—
Quercetin + Bromelain	—	1,000 to 2,000 mg/d (into 3 to 6 doses/d)	—	250 to 500 mg 1 to 2x/d	—	—
Pantothenic acid	—	500 mg 3x/d (after meals	—	50 mg 2 to 3x/d	—	—
Hydrochloric acid	—	1 or 2 after protein-based meals	—	—	—	—
★④ Antihistamines	—	OTC or Rx	—	OTC or Rx	—	OTC or Rx
Corticosteroid Nasal Spray	—	Rx	—	Rx	—	Rx
Allergy desensitization injections	Physician supervised					

A
L
L
E
R
G
I
E
S

O
N
L
Y

| | ADULTS | | CHILDREN (Over 3 yrs. of Age) | | PREGNANCY | |
	PREVENTIVE MAINTENANCE	TREATING ALLERGIES & ASTHMA	PREVENTION	TREATING ALLERGIES & ASTHMA	PREVENTION	TREATING ALLERGIES & ASTHMA
Anti-inflammatory agents (corticosteroids or cromolyn sodium	—	Rx	—	Rx	—	Rx
Bronchodilators (beta agonists and theophylline)	—	Rx	—	Rx	—	Rx
⭐5 Vitamin B-12	500 mcg 1x/d sublingually (under tongue)	500 mcg 2x/d	—	—	—	500 mcg 1x/d
Ginkgo biloba	—	40 mg of 24% standardized extract 3x/d	—	20 mg of 24% standardized extract 3x/d	—	—
Coleus forskholi	—	3 to 4 mg/d	—	—	—	—
N-acetylcysteine (NAC)	—	500 mg 2x/d	—	250 mg 2x/d	—	—
Ecomer (shark liver oil)	—	50 mg 3x/d	—	—	—	—
Flaxseed oil (or Omega-3 fatty acids)	2 Tbls/d	3 Tblsp/d	1 Tblsp/d	1 Tblsp/d	2 Tblsp/d	3 Tblsp/d

A S T H M A O N L Y ⭐6 (ASTHMA ONLY — rows from Vitamin B-12 through Ecomer)

*1 Use the higher dosages on days of higher stress, less sleep, more pollen, and increased pollution

*2 Can be used for both allergies and asthma; do not use with high blood pressure

*3 Do not use with high blood pressure or an enlarged prostate

*4 Allergies only—take these only during your allergy season; natural products may be taken with or without Rx's

*5 Magnesium, B-6, B-12, Ginkgo, and Coleus can be obtained in one product —Ventimax, made by CMC

*6 Asthma only—all of these can be taken together to control asthma, then gradually reduce Rx's while maintaining recommended dosages of natural products. This should be done under the supervision of a physician.

*7 Watch for low potassium with long-term use.

*8 Acidophilus can also be helpful for allergy and asthma treatment and prevention. Refer to "Sinusitis" Chart for dosages.

Both this chart and the "Sinusitis, Bronchitis, and Colds" Chart were created by Robert S. Ivker, D.O., Steve Morris, N.D., and Todd Nelson, N.D.

Chapter 9

CANDIDA

If you've been diligently doing all of the assigned "homework" from Chapter 8 and listening attentively to your body but the message is that there is still something basically wrong, then you may be one of the many millions of Americans who are unknowingly suffering from too much yeast.

Yeast is an integral part of life. It is a hardy fungus found in food, air, and on the exposed surfaces of most objects. There are more than 250 species of yeast organisms, and more than 150 of them can be found as harmless parasites in the human body. The most prevalent type of yeast found in and on our bodies is *Candida albicans*. It is an innocuous single-cell fungus and a normal inhabitant of our intestines primarily, and the mouth and vagina as well. Although not well documented, it is believed that its only function is to help absorb the B vitamins.

Candida is kept under control by the good bacteria that also make their home in the human gastrointestinal and genital tracts. A large percentage of the millions of these friendly bacteria are lactobacillus and bifidus. Similar to the bacteria in yogurt or in raw fermented foods, the lactobacilli make enzymes and vitamins, help fight undesirable bacteria, and lower cholesterol levels. While assisting us in keeping our bowel function and digestion normal, these friendly bacteria, also referred to as acidophilus bacteria, regard candida as their food. Since they are the chief "predator" of candida, they are critical to maintaining a "balance of nature" in our intestines. As long as this homeostatic relationship is maintained, candida poses no problem.

CAUSES

However, to an increasing extent massive overgrowth of candida is resulting in a condition medically known as candidiasis, candida-related complex, or candida toxicity syndrome. The most frequent *cause of this imbalance is the recurrent or extended use of antibiotics,* which kill the "good" bacteria along with those causing the infection for which the antibiotic is being taken. The more broad-spectrum the antibiotic, the broader the range of bacteria it will eliminate, therefore killing more of the lactobacilli. Millions of women are familiar with vaginal yeast infections, which develop when or just after using antibiotics. What I have repeatedly observed in my practice is that *the vast majority of people with chronic sinusitus, who have taken three or more ten-day to two-week courses of antibiotics within a six-month period, probably have some degree of candidiasis.* Since most antibiotics are given by mouth, the friendly bacteria of the intestines are particularly vulnerable to these medications.

Hormones, especially progesterone, and birth control pills can also contribute to causing candidiasis, which is why the overgrowth of candida is more prevalent in women than in men, children, or non-menstruating women. Progesterone, found in most birth control pills and also secreted at high levels during the ten to fourteen days prior to menstruation, has been shown to stimulate the growth of candida. The combination of high progesterone levels just prior to menstruation and an existing excess of candida can contribute to particularly severe symptoms of PMS (Premenstrual Syndrome). As you will see in Table 9-2, many of the symptoms of candidiasis are also present with PMS. Pregnancy is also favorable for candida, since it is accompanied by continuous high levels of progesterone.

Anything that weakens the immune system can contribute to

yeast overgrowth. Cortisone medications, such as prednisone and prednisolone, often used to treat chronic diseases such as asthma, arthritis, lupus, and colitis, are well-known immune system suppressants. They too have the potential for stimulating candidiasis, and can actually aggravate the disease the cortisone was treating. Chemotherapy and radiation treatments given to cancer patients can also weaken immunity and open the door to candida.

Any medication that can potentially cause gastrointestinal ulcerations or inflammation and weaken the lining of the gut can allow candida to gain a stronger and deeper foothold. These drugs might include aspirin, cortisone, and nonsteroidal anti-inflammatories such as Feldene, Naprosyn, Anaprox, Motrin, Advil, and Nuprin. Medicines given to ulcer patients, such as Tagamet or Zantac, can reduce acidity and raise pH levels high enough for yeast to grow. Candida thrive in a pH of 4 to 5, and normal stomach acidity is 2 to 3.

Environmental toxins and chemicals such as pesticides, herbicides, solvents, paints, formaldehyde, pentachlorophenol, combustion products of natural gas and coal (sulfur and nitrous oxide), petrochemicals (exhausts), and heavy metals such as lead, cadmium, arsenic, mercury, aluminum, and nickel can also weaken the immune system. People with occupational exposure to these substances are at highest risk for candidiasis, but as you've already learned, most of us in urban America live in such a toxic environment that we are all probably receiving significant exposure.

Table 9-1

Factors Tipping the Balance in Favor of Yeast

Antibiotics, primarily from medicines, also from commercial meats and poultry
Birth control pills
Pregnancy
Cortisone and other immunosuppressant drugs

Sugar
Alcohol
Typical American diet (high fat, high sugar, nutrient-poor)
Environmental chemicals
Chemotherapy and radiation
Free radicals
Food and other allergies
Malabsorption of nutrients
Deficiencies of hydrochloric acid, pancreatic enzymes, and bile
Undiagnosed hypothyroidism
Chronic viral infections
Occult parasitic infections, especially giardia and amoeba
Diabetes
Anti-inflammatory and other medications that produce gastrointestinal ulcerations
Acid antagonists (ulcer medications)
Major surgery
Physical trauma
Emotional trauma
Poor coping mechanisms to life's stresses
Diarrhea
Adrenal dysfunction—increased cortisol and decreased DHEA

(Reprinted with permission from *Optimal Wellness,* by Ralph T. Golan, M.D., Ballantine Books, 1995)

Other conditions that diminish immune function and can thereby potentially allow yeast overgrowth to occur are: allergies to inhalants, foods, or chemicals; viral infections such as Epstein-Barr virus (EBV), cytomegalovirus (CMV), human immunodeficiency virus (HIV), chronic or recurring flu illnesses; intestinal parasitic infections brought on by amoeba, giardia, or ascaris; hypothyroidism; nutrient deficiencies due to a poor diet or digestive problems (hydrochloric acid, pancreatic enzymes, and bile); major surgery; and emotional stress. The more severe the condition, the greater the potential for candidiasis.

Once the scale has been tipped and the overgrowth begins, it is fueled by the staple of the typical American diet—sugar. Like most of us, yeast consider sugar to be their favorite food. While candida thrive on it, sugar weakens our immune system. It decreases the ability of white blood cells, phagocytes in particular, to engulf unwanted organisms. It is therefore no surprise that diabetes, a chronic condition of high blood sugar, is also a major predisposing factor to candidiasis.

Obviously there are a multitude of causes that can contribute to creating the condition of candidiasis. In most instances, it is the combination of several factors occurring simultaneously that actually precipitates the overgrowth of yeast. Typically in patients with chronic sinusitis, the primary causes are: (1) repeated broad-spectrum antibiotics along with, (2) a sugar-filled diet, and (3) significant emotional stress. With many asthmatics, cortisone has been added to these three. As a general rule in medicine, as in life, there is rarely just one cause for anything. However, *in almost every instance of a particularly resistant case of chronic sinusitis, candida is a primary cause.* The same statement might also be true of asthma.

SYMPTOMS

Once the overgrowth occurs, the yeast invade the tissues of the gastrointestinal tract by growing in a plantlike form and sending roots into the walls of the small intestine. These roots can eventually bore holes in the intestinal wall, causing a condition known as "leaky gut syndrome." This means that the damage to the wall is allowing candida, bacteria, food, pollen, environmental pollutants, and other material to enter the bloodstream. It's almost as if your intestine has become a superabsorbent sponge. Candida often travel through the rectum and anus to the vagina and urinary tract and can subsequently enter the bloodstream via this more indirect route. Candida are then carried throughout the body and take up residence in those parts of the body with the most favorable environment for their growth—moist mucous membranes, especially those of the sinuses and lungs. In whatever tissue the candida have colonized, they cause inflammation and subsequent physical discomfort, such as sinus pain, muscle aches, joint pain, and itchy anus or vagina. There is still great controversy on this point: Are the candida organisms themselves traveling through the bloodstream and causing these symptoms throughout the body, or is it the toxins that have been released from candida?

As a result of widespread inflammation in the small bowel from the direct toxicity of candida, symptoms of the gastrointestinal tract are usually noticed first. Due to incomplete digestion and poor absorption of nutrients, these symptoms might include bloating, a feeling of fullness, diarrhea, constipation, alternating diarrhea and constipation, rectal itching, gas, and cramping. If the inflammation is severe and/or long-standing, it may be another contributing factor to causing leaky gut syndrome. As a result of this condition, large undigested particles of food, especially proteins, pass into the bloodstream and trigger multiple food allergies and sensitivities.

But the greatest health risks presented by candida result from the toxins they release (seventy-nine different ones have been identified), which can damage tissues directly or circulate throughout the bloodstream and cause problems in distant organs. These toxins can also significantly weaken the immune system by inhibiting the function of suppressor T-cells. These white blood cells, a type of lymphocyte, are responsible for modulating antibody production. When they are not working, there is a resulting excess of antibodies. The combination of this overabundance of antibodies along with the absorption of incompletely digested protein helps to explain the exaggerated sensitivities and *multiple adult-onset allergies,* both airborne and food, experienced by many people suffering "systemic" (whole body) candidiasis. The immune system sees the protein particles as antigens or foreign invaders of the body, and initiates a powerful "attack," resulting in an allergic reaction.

A yeast-impaired immune system also has less than the normal tolerance for ordinarily safe levels of common chemical odors such as gas and oil fumes, cleaning fluids, chlorine, perfume, etc.

An increasing number of people with candidiasis have become so allergic that almost every odor, all clothing except cotton, almost all foods, or anything in their immediate environment has become a major health problem. This condition has several names: multiple chemical sensitivity, environmental or ecological illness, or the universal reactor phenomenon. The immune system weakened by candida can also produce antibodies to the body's own tissues, especially the ovaries and thyroid, resulting in PMS and hypothyroid symptoms. These symptoms might include fatigue, irritability, sugar craving, headache, depression, and constipation.

One of the major toxins produced by yeast is acetaldehyde. Its multiple effects can be devastating. It is converted by the liver into alcohol, depleting the body of magnesium and potassium, reducing cell energy, and causing symptoms of intoxication—disorientation, dizziness, or mental confusion. The *spaciness* or *mental fog,* as it's often described by patients, is one of the most frequent symptoms of candidiasis. Patients relate a detached state of mind, poor concentration, faulty memory, and difficulty making decisions. The longer this condition persists, the more likely it is that depression will be added to the list of symptoms. The less oxygen in the body, the worse these symptoms are. Exercise, which supplies more oxygen, becomes more difficult to do because of this low-energy state. Energy is also depleted because acetaldehyde interferes with glucose metabolism—a key component of energy production. Along with other yeast toxins, acetaldehyde reduces the absorption of protein and minerals, which in turn diminishes the production of enzymes and hormones needed for energy. The combination of these multiple factors explains why *excessive fatigue* is the chief complaint of people with candidiasis. It usually comes on gradually but is most noticeable after a night's rest, after eating, and in mid- to late afternoon. If you eventually seek medical attention for extreme fatigue, a physical exam and lab tests will most likely be normal. You might even be told, "It's all in your head!" And if you weren't depressed before, you could begin to feel that way now.

The specific organ, tissue, or system damaged by candida will determine which symptoms occur. Table 9-2 is a comprehensive list of the possible symptoms of candidiasis. Many of them have other causes as well. However, if you have several, in addition to a history that is compatible with a yeast overgrowth, you can be relatively certain of the diagnosis.

Table 9-2

Possible Symptoms of Candidiasis

(I have underlined symptoms that are most common)

Brain and neurological
Fatigue and lethargy, lack of mental or physical stamina, depression, crying, mood swings, anxiety, nervousness, agitation, restlessness, grumpiness, explosive irritability, hostility, suicidal thoughts, loss of ability to concentrate, decreased intellectual functioning, behavior and learning problems, hyperactivity/poor attention span, tantrums, memory impairment, increasing lack of self-confidence, impaired ability to reason, "spacey" or unreal feeling, foggy/fuzzy/thick-minded, drunk feeling (without alcohol consumption), headaches (all varieties, including migraines), dizziness, lightheadedness, clumsiness/incoordination, shaking, insomnia, "schizophrenia," catatonia, autism, manic-depressive syndrome, psychosis, multiple sclerosis, myasthenia gravis.

Urogenital
Women: vaginal itching, burning, and/or discharge, vulvar itching and inflammation, vaginal or pelvic pain, painful intercourse, infertility. *Men:* impotence, recurrent prostatitis or inflammation of the prostate. *Both men and women:* recurrent urethritis/cystitis (bladder infection), bladder irritations, burning on urination, having to urinate too frequently, bladder "cramping," loss of sex drive.

Skin
Rough, dry, or scaly skin, acne, hives, generalized itching, eczema, chronic or recurrent fungal infections of the skin/nails, psoriasis, easy bruising, recurrent staph infections of the skin, folliculitis, rosacea, tingling, burning, numbness, and electrical feelings on the skin.

Ear
Ringing in the ear, stuffed or clogged ear, itching ears, recurrent ear infections, ear pain, diminished hearing.

Musculoskeletal
Arthritis, arthralgia, joint pain, joint stiffness, joint swelling, muscle pain/aching/discomfort, muscle weakness, muscle swelling, fatigue.

Gastrointestinal and bowel
Constipation, diarrhea, cramping, excessive gas, bloating and distention, intestinal "growling," mucousy or bloody stools, colitis, Crohn's disease, enteritis, irritable bowel syndrome, spastic colon, esophagitis, indigestion, heartburn, itchy anus, decreased appetite, oral thrush, canker sore, coated tongue, cracked/fissured tongue, chronic gum inflammation.

Respiratory
Chronic stuffy or runny nose, congested or allergic sinuses, chronic sneezing or coughing, asthma, shortness of breath/difficulty getting deep breath, recurrent or chronic sore throat, itchy throat, snoring, recurrent colds and flu, recurrent infections: sinusitis, tonsillitis, bronchitis, pneumonia, ear infections.

Menstrual/Female
Premenstrual symptoms: depression, emotional fragility, irritability, anxiety, fluid retention (including puffy face and fingers), breast tenderness, abdominal bloating, nausea, headaches, etc. Delayed periods, irregular periods, bleeding between periods, scanty or profuse bleeding, passing clots, painful periods, decreased libido (sexual desire), "endometriosis," infertility, miscarriages, fibrocystic breast disease, under-normal breast development.

Multiple allergies to foods; cravings for sweets, alcohol, bread, and cheese; intolerance or allergy to beverages and foods containing dietary yeasts and molds
Alcoholic beverages, aged cheeses, vinegar, soy sauce, peanuts, bread, brewer's yeast, B vitamins with yeast, mushrooms, bread and other yeast-raised baked items.

Chemical sensitivities
Cigarette smoke, exhaust fumes, perfumes, gasoline odor, new carpets, marking pens, paints, solvents, cleaning agents, etc.

Inhalant allergies

Mold, mildew (overall worsening condition in damp, cold season), "hay fever," dust, etc.

Heart/circulatory system

Rapid heartbeat, mitral valve prolapse, cold hands and feet.

Senses

Disturbances of smell, taste, vision and hearing (i.e., increased sensitivity to noise or light, deafness), salty or metallic taste, blurred vision, watery eyes.

Autoimmune

Rheumatoid arthritis, multiple diseases: sclerosis, systemic lupus erythematosis, myasthenia gravis, autoimmune hemolytic anemia, scleroderma, thyroiditis.

Other

Intolerance to heat and cold, hot and cold sweats, underweight, overweight, feeling sick all over, fluid retention/edema, anorexia nervosa, tendency to bleed easily/slow clotting.

This list is reprinted from *Optimal Wellness,* by Ralph T. Golan, M.D., Ballantine Books, 1995.

DIAGNOSIS

The most reliable way to make the diagnosis of candida is by compiling a thorough history and reviewing symptoms. If you are experiencing several of the possible symptoms and have a story compatible with causing candidiasis, there is no laboratory test that is as dependable as this combination for establishing the diagnosis. Further confirmation could be attained through the results of the treatment for yeast. In his book *The Yeast Connection,* William Crook, M.D., has formalized the symptom and history information into the Candida Questionnaire and Score Sheet, which can be ordered separately from Professional Books, P.O. Box 3494, Jackson, TN 38301. In his book, Dr. Crook says that yeast are especially apt to play a role in causing health problems in patients who:

1. Feel bad "all over," yet the cause can't be identified and treatment of many kinds hasn't helped.
2. Have taken prolonged courses of broad-spectrum antibiotics, including tetracycline, ampicillin, amoxicillin, Keflex, Ceclor, Septra, and Bactrim.
3. Have consumed diets containing a lot of yeast and sugar.
4. Crave sweets.
5. Crave other carbohydrates, especially breads and pizza.
6. Notice that sweets make symptoms worse or give a "pickup," followed by a "letdown."
7. Crave alcohol.
8. Have taken birth control pills, cortisone, or other corticosteroid drugs.
9. Have had multiple pregnancies.
10. Have been troubled by recurrent problems related to reproductive organs, including abdominal pain, vaginal infection or discomfort, premenstrual tension, menstrual irregularities, prostatitis, or impotence.
11. Are bothered by persistent or recurrent symptoms involving the digestive and nervous systems.
12. Have been bothered by athlete's foot, fungus infection of the nails, or jock itch.
13. Feel bad on damp days or in moldy places.
14. Are made ill when exposed to perfumes, tobacco smoke, and other chemicals.

The following is a modification of Dr. Crook's score sheet that can be used to reliably diagnose an overgrowth of candida.

Candida Questionnaire and Score Sheet

This questionnaire is designed for adults and the scoring system isn't appropriate for children. It lists factors in your medical history which promote the growth of candida albicans (Section A), and symptoms commonly found in individuals with yeast-connected illness (Sections B and C).

For each "Yes" answer in Section A, circle the point score in the box at the end of the section. Then move on to Sections B and C and score as directed.

Filling out and scoring the questionnaire should help you and your doctor evaluate the possible role of candida in contributing to your health problems. Yet it will not provide an automatic "Yes" or "No" answer.

SECTION A: HISTORY

Point Score

1. Have you taken tetracyclines (Symycin™, Panmycin™, Vibramycin™, Minocin™, etc) or other antibiotics for acne for one month or longer? 25

 • 2. Have you, at any time in your life, taken other "broad spectrum" antibiotics★ for respiratory, urinary or other infections for 2 months or longer or in shorter courses 4 or more times in a 1-year period? 20

 • 3. Have you taken a broad spectrum antibiotic★—even in a single course? 6

4. Have you, at any time in your life, been bothered by persistent prostatitis, vaginitis, or other problems affecting your reproductive organs? 25

5. Have you been pregnant
 • 2 or more times? 5
 1 time? 3

6. Have you taken birth control pills
 • For more than 2 years? 15
 For 6 months to 2 years? 8

7. Have you taken prednisone, Decadron or other cortisone-type drugs, by injection or inhalation
 • For more than 2 weeks? 15
 For 2 weeks or less? 6

8. Does exposure to perfumes, insecticides, fabric shop odors and other chemicals provoke
 Moderate to severe symptoms? 20
 Mild symptoms? 5

9. Are your symptoms worse on damp, muggy days or in moldy places? 20

10. Have you had athlete's foot, ring worm, jock itch or other chronic fungus infections of the skin or nails? Have such infections been

Severe or persistent?   20
• Mild to moderate?   10
• 11. Do you crave sugar?   10
12. Do you crave breads?   10
13. Do you crave alcoholic beverages?   10
• 14. Does tobacco smoke really bother you?   10

TOTAL SCORE, SECTION A _____ **9/**

*Including Keflex, ampicillin, amoxicillin, Ceclor, Bactrim, and Septra. Such antibiotics kill off "good germs" while they are killing off those which cause infection.

SECTION B: HISTORY   *Point Score*

For each of your symptoms, enter the appropriate figure in the point score column:

Occasional or mild   3 points
Frequent and/or moderately severe   6 points
Severe and/or disabling   9 points

Add total score and record it in the box at the end of this section.

Point Score

1. Fatigue or lethargy   _____ **6**
2. Feeling of being "drained"   _____ **6**
3. Poor memory or concentration   _____
4. Feeling "spacey" or "unreal"   _____ **3**
5. Depression   _____
6. Numbness, burning or tingling   _____
7. Muscle Aches   _____ **3**
8. Muscle weakness or paralysis   _____
9. Pain and/or swelling in joints   _____
10. Abdominal pain   _____ **6**
11. Constipation   _____
12. Diarrhea   _____ **3**
13. Bloating   _____
14. Troublesome vaginal discharge   _____
15. Persistent vaginal burning or itching   _____
16. Prostatitis   _____
17. Impotence   _____

18. Loss of sexual desire _____ 9
19. Endometriosis or infertility _____
20. Cramps and/or other menstrual irregularities _____
21. Premenstrual tension _____
22. Spots in front of the eyes _____ 3
23. Erratic vision _____

TOTAL SCORE, SECTION B _____ 39

SECTION C: OTHER SYMPTOMS

For each of your symptoms, enter the appropriate figure in the point score column:

Occasional or mild	1 points
Frequent and/or moderately severe	2 points
Severe and/or disabling	3 points

Add total score and record it in the box at the end of this section.

Point Score

1. Drowsiness _____ 1
2. Irritability or jitteriness _____
3. Incoordination _____
4. Inability to concentrate _____
5. Frequent mood swings _____
6. Headache _____ 1
7. Dizziness/loss of balance _____
8. Pressure above ears, feeling of head swelling and tingling _____
9. Itching _____
10. Other rashes _____ 2
11. Heartburn _____
12. Indigestion _____
13. Belching and intestinal gas _____ 1
14. Mucous in stools _____ 2
15. Hemorrhoids _____
16. Dry mouth _____
17. Rash or blisters in mouth _____
18. Bad breath _____
19. Joint swelling or arthritis _____
20. Nasal congestion or discharge _____
21. Postnasal drip _____ 1

22. Nasal itching   *1*
23. Sore or dry throat   *1*
24. Cough   *2*
25. Pain or tightness in chest
26. Wheezing or shortness of breath   *2*
27. Urinary urgency or frequency
28. Burning on urination
29. Failing vision
30. Burning or tearing of eyes
31. Recurrent infections or fluid in ears
32. Ear pain or deafness

TOTAL SCORE, SECTION C   *15*

TOTAL SCORE, SECTION A   *91*

TOTAL SCORE, SECTION B   *39*

GRAND TOTAL SCORE   *135*

The Grand Total Score will help you and your doctor decide if your health problems are yeast-connected. Scores in women will run higher as 7 items in the questionnaire apply exclusively to women, while only 2 apply exclusively to men.

If your score is:	Symptoms are:
180 (women)	Almost Certainly
140 (men)	Yeast Connected
120 (women)	Probably
80 (men)	Yeast connected
60 (women)	Possibly
40 (men)	Yeast Connected
Less than	
60 (women)	Probably Not
40 (men)	Yeast Connected

Much of the original research on candida was performed by C. Orian Truss, M.D., who wrote *The Missing Diagnosis*. In that book he states that the diagnosis of systemic candidiasis should be suspected in any individual with chronic sinus and upper respiratory conditions and allergies, runny nose, postnasal drip, mucus in the throat, itchy ears, or chronic sore throat.

The current laboratory tests that have been most often used to diagnose candida are:

Cultures—of stool primarily, but also vaginal, nasal, throat, and skin. Cultures are often unreliable because they will show no yeast when in fact yeast are present. This occurs because candida does not grow in the bowel in a uniform fashion, like rust around a pipe. The greatest value of the stool test is to determine the amount of good bacteria. If the lactobacilli are missing, then we know candida has an excellent chance of growing. Cultures should be done in combination with blood tests to compensate for false negative results.

Candida antigen titer test—a blood test to determine if yeast antigens or toxins are present. Although better than the stool culture, there can also be false negatives when the toxins are present but bound to an antibody in an antigen/antibody complex, which the test does not detect.

Candida antibodies and immune complexes—measures the level of antibodies your immune system cells have made to fight candida. This method of diagnosis is also less than ideal. Since the body normally has some candida antibodies, high counts don't always mean a current yeast overgrowth, interpretation of the results can be difficult, and the test is expensive.

Due to their unreliability, these laboratory tests have not met the current high scientific standards expected for medical diagnosis. It is primarily for this reason that the majority of physicians fail to recognize the existence of systemic candidiasis, and many have become antagonistic even to the suggestion of that diagnosis. Unfortunately, this lack of acknowledgment prevents most physicians from ever treating the condition. Although they're not perfect, these tests can still be helpful in the diagnosis of candida. Ultimately, regardless of the test results, a trial candida treatment program has been the best diagnostic test we've had. If there's a definite improvement in your symptoms within four weeks or even sooner, then you probably have candidiasis.

More than two years ago I had the opportunity of working with Claude Selitrennikoff, Ph.D., a professor of cell biology at the University of Colorado School of Medicine, and one of the world's foremost authorities on the subject of candida. For more than fifteen years, the primary mission of his research had been the development of novel antifungal drugs. While in the course of helping him treat his own candidiasis, I discussed the diagnostic dilemma confronting the medical community and the burgeoning ranks of undiagnosed patients suffering with this condition. As a result, he has developed a candida antigen test called the Sinus Survival Candidetect. Dr. Selitrennikoff observed that when candida cells divide, they release a water-soluble antigen, called beta-glucan. His test utilizes an antibody that is specific for and will quantitate the amount of beta-glucan in both urine and blood. Beta-glucan can *only* be present due to yeast cell division. The Candidetect is much more sensitive and reliable than current diagnostic tests. It is also simpler, more convenient, and less expensive. The test is designed to be performed at home with either urine (similar to home pregnancy tests) or a finger stab (similar to self-testing of diabetics for blood glucose), and will yield quantitative results within twenty minutes. People who suspect candidiasis can make a definitive diagnosis on their own and monitor the progress of their treatment program. Because of the prevalence of yeast overgrowth in causing chronic sinusitis, this test will become an integral part of the Sinus Survival Program. It is not yet available for sale, but pending FDA approval is expected to be sometime in 1996.

TREATMENT

Although similar in its holistic scope, the comprehensive treatment program for systemic candidiasis is more challenging than the regimen for simple chronic sinusitis (i.e., without candida). Treatment depends upon the degree of yeast overgrowth and to what extent immune function has been diminished. If yeast symptoms are confined only to the gastrointestinal tract or vagina, the program is shorter and much less involved than if the yeast toxins have spread throughout the body and are causing recurrent sinus infections along with other problems. In the latter case, which is most often the situation with my patients, it can take from six to nine months to cure candidiasis.

The treatment program for systemic candidiasis consists of four components, and for the best results you should start with parts I and II before progressing to III and IV:

I. Kill the overgrowth of candida.
II. Eliminate the fuel for the growth of candida through diet.
III. Restore normal bacterial flora in the bowel.
IV. Strengthen the immune system.

I. The most effective means of killing candida is through the use of the prescription antifungal drugs Nizoral, Diflucan, and Sporonox. Although they're all expensive (200mg of Diflucan can cost as much as $13 per tablet; 200mg of Nizoral averages about $3) and have potentially harmful side effects, nothing else works as well. They're usually prescribed at 200mg per day for at least one month. Diflucan is recommended daily for six weeks, and I will often reduce Nizoral to one every other day for a second month. Many physicians are reluctant to prescribe these, especially Nizoral, because of possible liver toxicity. During the five years that I have been prescribing it, I have seen only two patients develop the symptoms of hepatitis (inflammation of the liver) from Nizoral, and both resolved quickly after stopping the drug. A blood test for liver enzymes before starting on Nizoral would be helpful in minimizing this risk, as well as taking silymarin (milk-thistle extract), which protects the liver. A more probable side effect in using these drugs is die-off, or the "Herxheimer reaction," which usually occurs during the first one to two weeks of treatment. These medications are so powerful in killing yeast that as the organisms die they release a "flood" of toxins into the bloodstream that can cause fatigue, headaches, nausea, loose stools, flulike aches and pains, and any other symptom that yeast are known to produce. Distilled water, both drunk and used as an enema, vitamin C, and ibuprofen can all help to relieve these die-off symptoms. Although it's possible that for a short time you might feel worse than you did before, you might also choose to look at the "regression" resulting from die-off as a confirmation of your diagnosis of candida, as well as a hopeful sign that you are eliminating yeast and will be feeling much better very soon. The other prescription drug that's been around far longer than the others I've mentioned is Nystatin, available in tablets and powder. It kills candida very well in the bowel, but is ineffective for the rest of the body.

If you are not able to obtain or cannot take a prescription antifungal drug, there are other available options that work, although they are not quite as effective in quickly reducing candida. Three homeopathic remedies that I'm familiar with are Aqua Flora and Candida-Away (available in health-food stores) and Mycocan Combo, available only through health care practitioners. I've used Mycocan with many patients and have seen good results. For a stronger combination, these homeopathics can also be used in conjunction with Nystatin. There are a variety of products available in health food stores that can help to eliminate candida. Most contain caprylic acid, garlic, pau d'arco, and other herbs that act directly on candida or indirectly by strengthening the immune system. Some of these anti-yeast products that you're likely to find in health food stores are Yeast Fighters, Candida Cleanse, Cand-Ex, Caprystatin Yeast Defense, and Cantrol. There is some evidence that candida will develop a resistance to each of these substances after using them for about seven days. Therefore, I recommend rotating four or five of these and using each one for less than a week, maintaining the rotation for a total of three months. These anti-yeast products may also be used following drug therapy as a method of preventing candida from "rebounding."

Another product that I always use in my practice to kill candida is Flora Balance. It is a unique strain of bacteria called Bacillus laterosporus B.O.D. that is available in health food stores, or through physicians as Latero-Flora. It has been tested extensively and found to be extremely effective for gastrointestinal dysfunction, food sensitivities, and candidiasis. It is suggested that two capsules be taken twenty minutes before breakfast. I usually continue that dose for about two months before reducing it to one daily capsule for another one to two months.

An herbal combination (made up of more than twenty herbs) that I frequently use as part of my candida elimination program is Intestinalis. It is an excellent remedy for any intestinal infection. In addition to treating candida, it can be used to treat or even prevent giardia, a parasite frequently found in untreated water, and traveler's diarrhea. Two years ago, a woman I was treating for chronic sinusitis and candidiasis went on a group tour to Egypt. Upon her return she was so pleased to report to me that she was the only member of the forty-person group who did not get diarrhea. I'm certain that she was also the only one on the tour taking Intestinalis every day.

In recent years there have been reports of dramatic results in eliminating candida using 35 percent food-grade hydrogen peroxide. (Store-bought hydrogen peroxide is a 3 percent solution.) It can be taken orally or intravenously. I have had no personal experience with this method, but I have read about Dr. Kurt Donsbach's success using this treatment at his holistic center, Hospital Santa Monica in Rosarito Beach, Baja California, Mexico.

The average American diet can cause a thick coat of mucus and impacted food residue to form on the walls of the large intestine. Not only can this encrusted matter affect colon function and contribute to disease by preventing absorption of vital nutrients, it also provides an ideal environment for yeast to thrive. That's why colonic treatments provide another rapid method of removing excess candida from the bowel as well as mitigating die-off effects. Much more effective than an enema, they are best done on a weekly basis in conjunction with taking an antifungal drug. They can cleanse the bowel of candida, toxins, and dead yeast organisms, while also helping the inflamed lining of the bowel to begin the healing process. These treatments need to be performed by trained practitioners, and in most cities they are not that easy to find. Look for them through the office of a chiropractor or naturopath.

Although not as fast (it can take several months), it is possible to clean the colon by following a candida-control diet, drinking plenty of water, getting regular exercise, taking caprylic acid to kill candida, and using two natural agents that eliminate colon toxicity—psyllium and bentonite. Mix one heaping teaspoon of psyllium plus two tablespoons of liquid bentonite with 8 to 10 ounces of water or diluted juice twice a day (morning and night). If there is bloating, cut the above dosages in half but still take it two times a day.

II. Eliminating the fuel for candida through diet, while at the same time strengthening your immune system, is the foundation of any treatment program. Since each of us has a unique body chemistry, no two candida-control diets will be exactly the same. Also, every physician who treats candidiasis has somewhat different dietary recommendations. But there are some basic principles that apply to almost anyone:

1. The diet consists primarily of protein and fresh vegetables and a limited amount of complex carbohydrates and fat-containing foods, along with a small amount of fresh fruit.
2. Sugar and concentrated sweets are always to be avoided.
3. Three to six months is a minimum time frame for maintaining the diet, although it can be less restrictive the longer you're on it.
4. It's best to rotate the acceptable foods and not eat a particular food more than once every three or four days.
5. Changing one's diet can be a challenge. The more involved you are in the process—planning, shopping, and cooking—the easier and more rewarding it will be.

The following diet is a composite from the two naturopathic physicians with whom I work closely on treating candida, Todd

Nelson and Sylvia Flesner, and my holistic medical colleague Ralph Golan, M.D.

Foods to Include

*Vegetables:*eat freely; 50 to 60 percent of total diet; raw or lightly steamed; organic and clean (wash well); high-water content and low-starch vegetables are best:

- green leafy: all lettuce, spinach, parsley, cabbage, kale, collard greens, watercress, beet greens, mustard greens, bok choy, sprouts;
- other low-starch vegetables: celery, zucchini, summer squash, crookneck squash, green beans, broccoli, cauliflower, brussels sprouts, radish, bell pepper (green, red, yellow), asparagus, cucumber, tomato, onion, leek, garlic, kohlrabi;
- moderately low starch: carrot, beet, rutabaga, turnip, parsnip, eggplant, artichoke, avocado, water chestnuts, peas (green, snow peas), okra.

Protein: eat freely; meats should be antibiotic and hormone free; fish should be fresh deep-water ocean fish; seeds and nuts should be raw organic. Acceptable proteins include: fish, canned fish—salmon and tuna (okay occasionally), turkey, ground turkey, chicken, lamb, wild game, cornish hen, eggs (limit two to four per week), seeds and nuts—almonds, cashews, pecans, filberts, pine nuts, brazil nuts, walnuts, pistachios, sunflower seeds, sesame seeds (raw or dry roasted), pumpkin seeds.

Complex Carbohydrates: includes starchy vegetables, legumes (introduce after the first twenty-one days), and whole grains; eat only enough to maintain your energy (try to limit to one serving a day or less); restriction varies according to food allergy, which can be determined with food rotation.

- starchy vegetables: potatoes, sweet potatoes, yams, winter squash (acorn, butternut), pumpkin;

- legumes: lentils, split peas, black-eyed peas, beans (kidney, garbanzo, black, navy, pinto, lima, aduki);
- whole grains: sprouted or cooked, such as rice; organic and clean; available in bulk at health food stores; rotate grains every four days; tasty as breakfast cereals, in salads and soups, in casseroles and stirfrys; store away from light and heat in airtight containers; non-gluten grains are best—brown rice, millet, quinoa, and amaranth; other whole grains that should be eaten in only limited amounts include barley, spelt, wild rice, corn, buckwheat, oats, cornmeal, popcorn, bulgur, and couscous.

Flaxseed Oil: 1 to 2 tablespoons daily; use on grains or vegetables, or as a salad dressing; do *not* heat or cook with; keep refrigerated and away from light; other acceptable oils (cold pressed)—linseed, walnut, safflower, sunflower, soy.

Fruits: Introduce fruits into your diet slowly, limiting yourself to one serving per day until you are sure they do not make your symptoms worse. Start with melons, berries—blueberries, raspberries, huckleberries, blackberries, lemon and grapefruit (only after first twenty-one days of the diet); then choose from among most other fresh fruits, all of which are generally sweeter than the first group. These include apple, pear, peach, orange, nectarine, apricot, cherry, and pineapple. Grapefruit juice is okay, but other fruit juices should be very diluted, at least 1:1 with water. Freshly squeezed is best. Avoid full-strength fruit juices, canned fruit juices, and all dried fruits.

Yeast and Mold-Containing Foods: these are allowable only if you're not allergic. However, I would introduce them very gradually (eat a particular food no more than once every three to four days) and not begin until you have been on the diet for at least three weeks. These foods include: enriched flour; fermented dairy products such as yogurt, kefir, buttermilk, low-fat cottage cheese, and sour cream; fermented foods such as tofu, tempeh, miso, soy sauce; raw almond butter and raw sesame tahini.

Foods to Avoid

- refined sugar and sugar-containing foods: cakes, cookies, candy, doughnuts, pastries, ice cream, pudding, soft drinks, pies, etc.; anything containing sucrose (table sugar), fructose, maltose, lactose, glucose, dextrose, corn sweetener, corn syrup, sorbitol, and manitol; honey; molasses; maple syrup; date sugar; barley malt; rice syrup; Nutra Sweet; and saccharine; table salt (contains 50 percent sugar; use sea salt).

  Chromium picolinate, 200mcg 2×/day; biotin, 500–1,000mcg 2×/day; and a yeast-free B-complex, 50mg 2×/day can help to diminish sugar cravings, although four days without any sugar will usually eliminate this craving.
- milk and dairy products—all cheeses; (unsweetened soy milk is okay and so is butter, but not in excess);
- bread and other yeast-raised baked items, including cakes, cookies, and crackers; whole grain cereals; pastas; tortillas; waffles; and muffins;
- beef and pork;
- mushrooms—all types;
- rye and wheat (avoid for first three weeks);
- grapes, plums, bananas, dried fruit, canned fruit, and canned vegetables;
- alcoholic beverages;
- caffeine—both tea and coffee (herbal tea is okay);
- white or refined flour products, packaged/processed and refined foods;
- fried foods, fast foods, sausage, and hot dogs;
- vinegar, mustard, ketchup, sauerkraut, olives, and pickles;
- margarine, preservatives (check frozen vegetables), artificial sweeteners;
- refined and hydrogenated oils;
- leftovers—freeze them for a later date.

This diet is meant to be a guide. The responses to it will vary greatly depending upon the severity of the candidiasis, food allergies, and the type of medication (if any) you're taking to eliminate candida. The majority of people who closely adhere to it will experience a significant improvement within one month. But suppose you've been following it for three to four weeks in addition to taking medication and you've seen no improvement. Then I'd recommend going back to the basic vegetable (low starch) and protein diet and be suspicious of food allergy. The food you're allergic to is often something you eat every day and have developed a craving for. If you reintroduce new foods very gradually, every three to four days, then you should be able to detect the offending food from the symptoms that arise after eating it.

Initially many people complain, "There's nothing to eat on this diet," and it's not unusual to lose eight to ten pounds during the first month. However, there are in fact a multitude of nutritious and tasty choices, and the weight loss will usually subside. A key factor in successfully maintaining the diet lies in finding some recipes that you like. Candida cookbooks are relatively easy to locate in most health food stores. Gail Burton's *Candida Control Cookbook,* Dr. Crook's *The Yeast Connection Cook Book,* and Vicki Glassburn's *Who Killed Candida?* are all excellent resources. The menu and recipe suggestions that follow have been provided by Todd Nelson, N.D., and his assistant, Rose Weber.

Menu Suggestions for a Candida Hypo-Allergenic Diet

★ = recipe included
★★ = at health food store

Breakfast Suggestions
- non-gluten whole grain porridge★
- non-gluten whole grain hot cereal★
- mochi waffle★★

- ¹/₂ baked acorn squash★
- baked sweet potatoes
- new red potatoes and steamed vegetables
- 12 raw almonds, walnuts, filberts, pecans, or pine nuts
- small handful of raw sunflower seeds or pumpkin seeds
- ground raw sesame or flaxseeds sprinkled on hot cereal
- nut butter or nut milk★
- steamed vegetables
- eggs

Lunch Suggestions
Protein/Vegetable Combinations

- fresh green salad with raw nuts or seeds
- fresh green salad with turkey, fish, lamb, beef, or chicken
- fresh green salad with sprouted beans or cooked beans
- steamed vegetables sprinkled with ground-up raw nuts or seeds
- steamed vegetables and an animal protein
- steamed vegetables or salad and bean, lentil, or pea soup★
- vegetable and nut stirfry (no rice)
- vegetable and animal protein stirfry (no rice)
- fresh tuna salad with no mayo
- vegetable and animal protein soup
- vegetable and bean soup
- vegetable soup or stew★
- fresh vegetable sticks and nut butter for dip
- fresh vegetables and hummus for dip★★
- steamed asparagus wrapped in thinly sliced turkey breast
- turkey or chicken drumsticks and vegetables

Dinner Suggestions
Complex Carbohydrate/Vegetable Combinations

- vegetable and non-gluten whole grain casserole★
- vegetable and non-gluten whole grain salad★
- vegetable and non-gluten whole grain soup★
- rice paper spring rolls with no sauce★★
- vegetable nori rolls with no mustard★★

- steamed vegetables or green salad with new red potatoes
- vegetables and baked squash or sweet potatoes
- vegetables with beans and rice
- vegetable stirfry with a non-gluten whole grain
- non-gluten pasta salad
- non-gluten pasta with dairy-free pesto sauce★★ and vegetables
- mashed potatoes and vegetables with flax oil
- stuffed peppers with a non-gluten whole grain and vegetables★
- dairy-free new red potato salad with vegetables
- vegetable sandwich on a non-gluten whole grain bread★

Beverages
- herb teas★★
- fresh organic vegetable juice diluted 50 percent★★ (Rainbow Brand–carrot, "nature's garden," or beet combination)
- pure water
- fresh grated gingerroot tea

Flavorings
- flax oil for salad dressings or in place of butter on steamed vegetables or cooked grains
- cold-pressed olive oil or sesame oil (Omega Nutrition)
- Quick-Sip by Bernard Jensen as a salt substitute (found in most health food stores)
- fresh lemon, lime, or grapefruit juice in dressings or on steamed vegetables
- fresh herbs: cilantro, mint, basil, dill, parsely, or rosemary to flavor salads and grains
- fresh spices★★ (avoid salt and black pepper)
- use butter instead of margarine
- garlic (great for candida diets)
- gingerroot
- nut butter for sauces and dressings
- Bragg Liquid Aminos (a non-fermented soy sauce)
- seasalt (use sparingly)

Snack Suggestions
- organic vegetable sticks
- raw organic almonds, walnuts, filberts, pine nuts, sunflower seeds, or pumpkin seeds
- rice cakes
- rice cakes with raw nut butter
- nut milk★
- amasake or rice milk★★
- non-gluten or whole grain pasta
- plain mochi (snack bread made with brown rice)★★
- hummus★★
- nori roll★★
- sweet potatoes
- baked acorn squash

Recipes for a Candida Hypo-Allergenic Diet
Breakfast Recipes

WHOLE GRAIN PORRIDGE
Use leftover (already cooked) non-gluten grains: brown rice, millet, amaranth, or quinoa. Place the cold grain in the blender with water, juice, rice milk, or nut milk. The amount of liquid determines how thick the porridge will be. Blend together to desired consistency. Heat the porridge. Add flax oil to taste. Be creative and try other flavorings such as cinnamon, almond butter, banana, ground flaxseeds, raisins, apple sauce, or almond slivers. No two porridges are alike.

WHOLE GRAIN HOT CEREAL
If you like Cream of Wheat, why not try Cream of Millet, Cream of Amaranth, or Cream of Quinoa? Pick any non-gluten grain and grind up 1/2 cup in a coffee grinder. Add the grain very gradually to 1 1/2 cups boiling water or apple juice, stirring constantly. Simmer for five minutes. Top it off with nut milk and flax oil. Also try nuts and seeds, cinnamon, apple sauce, or banana slices. Quick, easy, and yummmmmy!

Nut Milk

Place ¹/₂ cup raw almonds, sunflower seeds, sesame seeds, or cashews and two cups of water in the blender. Blend until smooth and creamy. Strain milk through a cheesecloth. Flavor with cinnamon. Delicious hot or cold, and a great milk substitute for baking.

Sprouted Grains

Soak a non–gluten grain for 12–24 hours, rinsing twice daily until tiny, ¹/₄-inch sprouts begin to appear. At this point, spread the sprouts on a towel and allow to dry for 1 to 4 hours. Do not allow them to wither and harden. Place in refrigerator and they will last three to ten days. To serve, warm the sprouts very carefully in a pan with melted butter or soak in hot tap water for a minute or so. Eat them for breakfast or in place of cooked grains at other meals.

Sprouts are high in fiber; the enzymes in the grains have not been destroyed by heat, and they are often less allergenic than cooked grains.

Acorn Squash

Cut squash in half and steam facedown for 20 to 30 minutes. Set in an oven dish and fill with 1 teaspoon butter. Place in 350-degree oven for 10 minutes. Also delicious with flax oil, but do not add until after baking. (Avoid maple syrup or honey.)

Lunch and/or Dinner Recipes

Bieler's Broth

Steam 2 medium zucchini, a handful of green beans, and 2 stalks of celery until they are very soft. Place the vegetables and the steaming water in the blender and blend for 1 to 2 minutes until smooth. Add fresh parsley and serve hot.

Vegetable Soup

In a large saucepan, sauté diced celery, carrot, zucchini, broccoli, cauliflower, cabbage, onion, and garlic in a little pure water.

Cover with water and add 1 tablespoon oregano, 1 tablespoon basil, and cayenne to taste. Simmer 1/2 hour. Serve, then add Quick-Sip to taste. Also try this soup with diced new red potatoes or sweet potatoes.

Split Pea Soup
Dice and sauté carrots, celery, and onion. Boil 1 cup green split peas in 1/2 to 1 quart water. Add vegetables after 20 minutes. Add 1/4 teaspoon thyme.

Clean Casserole
Steam zucchini and celery for 5 minutes. Turn off burner, add a good portion of mung bean sprouts, and let sit for 5 minutes. Place 1/2 inch of cooked rice in bottom of buttered casserole dish. Pour vegetables on top of rice and sprinkle with sunflower seeds. Bake at 350 degrees for 20 minutes. Allow to cool slightly, then add 1 to 2 tablespoons butter or flax oil, and sprinkle with Quick-Sip.

Curry Rice
Sauté mushrooms, onion, and green peppers in butter. Add cooked brown rice, a little Quick-Sip, and curry powder to taste. Garnish with fresh chopped parsley. Serve with sautéed vegetables and a side of coconut.

Quinoa Salad
   1 3/4 cups pure water
   1 cup quinoa, rinsed 2 or 3 times
   1/2 cup finely diced cucumber or celery
   4 stems finely diced green onion
   1/4 cup finely diced fresh cilantro
   3 tablespoons fresh lime juice
   2 tablespoons flax oil
   Sea salt to taste
   Cayenne pepper to taste

Bring water to a boil in a 1-quart pot, then add quinoa. Reduce heat and simmer, covered, for 15 minutes, stirring occasionally until grain is tender. Remove from heat and let cool, uncovered. Toss cucumber, green onion, and cilantro with cooked quinoa. Combine the lime juice, oil, salt, and cayenne, and add to quinoa. Stir thoroughly with a fork to coat the grains and vegetables.

VEGGIE SANDWICH

Pile high on a non-gluten bread any or all of the following: grated carrot, cucumber, green pepper, onion, sprouts, lettuce, avocado. Sprinkle with your favorite herbs and spices.

ROSE'S SAUCE

Mix together 1–2 tablespoons flax oil, 1–2 tablespoons raw sesame tahini, 2 teaspoons Quick-Sip, and fresh lemon juice to taste. Top steamed vegetables (cabbage, onion, zucchini, and red pepper make a great combination) and wild rice. Serve hot. This also makes a great salad dressing if you decrease the tahini and increase the lemon juice. Add your favorite herbs and spices.

III. The best way to restore normal bacterial flora in the bowel is through the administration of "acidophilus bacteria." This should be done after phase I and during phase II (diet) of the treatment program. The good bacteria cannot grow back fully until the yeast overgrowth in the bowel has been greatly diminished. A reasonable time to begin phase III is about six weeks into the program.

The friendly intestinal bacteria can be restored through a multitude of lactobacillus acidophilus and bifidus products available in health food stores. These can be found in liquids, powders, capsules, and tablets. There are new and better strains being developed on a regular basis, with a wide variety of potency. While there are many brands of acidophilus and bifidus sold in health food stores, most of these actually contain only a small amount of *living* organisms because these products lack the nutrients necessary for survival. Even freeze-dried types usually contain insufficient amounts of acidophilus at the time of use, despite the billions-of-organisms-per-gram content at the time of bottling. To assure potency, follow these guidelines:

1. Buy only refrigerated brands that clearly state an expiration date between one and ten months from the date the item is purchased.

2. Buy either liquid cultures (such as yogurt culture) or powdered forms containing whey (dairy) or non-dairy varieties. Lactobacilli are living organisms and only these forms provide an ample food supply with which to sustain the fragile acidophilus bacteria.

Be aware that many yogurt products do not contain a high amount of viable organisms by the time they reach the consumer. This is especially true of highly processed ones, or those with many additional ingredients. People who are sensitive to dairy products, as well as those with chronic respiratory disease, should not use yogurt as a consistent source of friendly bacteria. Remember to avoid those brands of yogurt that have added sweeteners.

IV. Strengthening the immune system is a vital aspect of treating candidiasis. Phases I, II, and III can all contribute in varying degrees to a stronger immune system. In addition to the complete vitamin, mineral, and herbal regimen described in Chapter 8, I recommend:

- biotin, 300 to 1,000mcg 3×/day;
- flaxseed oil (already a part of the candida diet) or other essential fatty acids found in primrose or black currant oils;
- amino acid supplements;
- adrenal-enhancing supplements (I use a product called Adrenal Complex available only through practitioners).

The remainder of the physical health recommendations in Chapter 8—a whole-foods diet (not as restrictive as the candida diet), adequate water intake, and regular exercise—as well as the guidelines concerning mental, emotional, social, and spiritual health found in chapters 10 through 13 will all contribute to a powerful immune system.

If you are highly suspicious that you have candidiasis, have followed this treatment plan for one to three months, and still experience little or no improvement, there are other options available to you. If you have not already done so, I recommend consulting with your physician about the possibility of taking one of the anti-fungal prescription drugs—Nizoral, Diflucan, or Sporonox. If you've already completed a full course of one of these medications with no improvement, then I'd be most suspicious of food allergy and leaky gut syndrome. This condition can take close to a year to completely resolve, even using some of the new and highly effective dietary supplements formulated to treat this challenging problem. Ultra Clear® and Clear Tox are the products I've used for leaky gut syndrome with excellent results. The former was formulated and developed by Jeffrey S. Bland, Ph.D., a clinical biochemist and internationally known authority on therapeutic nutrition. They help to detoxify the body, feed the good bacteria, and assist in healing the "leaky" intestinal lining. Clear Tox is available through some health food stores and Klabin Marketing.

The other possible but less likely coexisting conditions that might be preventing improvement are: intestinal parasites (especially giardia), inhalant mold allergy, hypochlorhydria, pancreatic enzyme deficiency, helicobacter pylori, hypothyroidism, adrenal exhaustion, chronic viral infections/chronic fatigue syndrome, chemical injury or hypersensitivity, heavy metal poisoning (especially mercury toxicity from silver mercury amalgam dental fillings), and hormone hypersensitivity (particularly to progesterone). Obviously you will need to work with your physician to investigate these possible diagnoses. You may also be getting re-infected with candida from your regular sexual partner. Men, particularly, may transmit candida without being symptomatic themselves, although it is possible for women to be the asymptomatic transmitters.

You will know when you have completely recovered from

candidiasis because you'll probably feel better than you have in years. You might want to review your initial list of symptoms just to make sure, but most people have no trouble determining that the candida overgrowth is resolved. Don't allow this hard-earned victory over a tenacious foe to be short-lived. Try to maintain a healthy diet without reverting back to excess sugar and alcohol. Remember: *moderation*. Continue to nurture yourself in body, mind, and spirit and your immune system will afford you excellent health with no concern about the recurrence of candida.

Chapter 10

MENTAL HEALTH

The breadth of the term *mental health* is so great it almost defies definition. In my opinion, true mental health means that you are both aware of and are practicing your gifts and special talents; recognizing the extent to which your thoughts, beliefs, attitudes, and mental pictures limit or expand your potential to enjoy life; learning that you always have choices; attaining a high degree of clarity regarding your priorities, values, and goals; working at a job that you enjoy; and incorporating humor, forgiveness, gratitude, and hope into your life. The end result is a condition that combines peace of mind with living your dreams.

It is not within the scope of this book to explore any of these areas in great depth. I would, however, like you to become more aware of how your mental health affects your physical health, and to learn some simple things that will help you attain a greater degree of mental fitness.

BELIEFS, AFFIRMATIONS, GOALS, AND NLP

Most patients who come to see me have already sought help from one or even several physicians. Their doctors have told them, "You're going to have to live with your sinus problem"; "You have six months left to live with that cancer"; "Your back/ sinus/knee requires surgery"; or "There's nothing more that can be done for it" (the majority of diseases). These statements are, however, only beliefs. The beliefs are based on the limitations of modern medical science, a highly scientific and technologically advanced approach to the treatment of disease, and they are delivered to the patient by a highly educated individual in a society that defers to expertise. These pronouncements, which are in some cases death sentences, are quickly accepted by most patients and become a part of their own belief system. The vast majority of people with terminal diseases who accept whatever their doctors tell them (these patients are called "compliant") die very close to the predicted time. Patients who challenge prognoses tend to live longer. In *Love, Medicine and Miracles,* Bernie Siegel, M.D., vividly describes how the beliefs and attitudes of many of his cancer patients affected the outcome of their disease.

Most of the beliefs held by Americans have been defined by the standards, or norms, of our society, but how well does the norm fit you, a unique individual? If all of us attempted to conform, the world would be a boring place, devoid of creativity and innovation. We certainly wouldn't be enjoying the ease of living that technology has provided us were it not for the adventuresome few who deviated from the conventional belief system.

Unfortunately, in every culture there is great pressure to conform. It isn't easy, to say the least, to hold beliefs that run counter to prevalent attitudes. Society, friends, and family all tell us we have strayed with phrases such as "you should," "you ought to," or—if your belief has caused them a lot of discomfort —"you're crazy!" Most of the time we respond to this pressure by giving up our unreasonable, or even outrageous, belief. Ultimately, all of us would prefer to be accepted and loved by others; besides, we tell ourselves, "it wasn't that big a deal anyway."

Your belief system has a profound impact on your life: what you eat and think, how you dress and behave, what you do for a living, how you spend your leisure time, what your values and goals are, and how you define health and quality of life. It also determines the nature of the silent messages you give yourself every day. All of us talk to ourselves, and this internal dialogue has a great deal to do with our state of mental health. These messages might be generally self-critical ("You stupid . . ."; "Why did you say that?"; "Why did you do that?"; "How could you . . . ?"; "You should've/could've . . ."); or they might be accepting and supportive ("Good job!"; "That's fine"; "You did the best you could"). Almost all of my patients are very hard on themselves. They are self-critical and put themselves under a great deal of unnecessary pressure.

As human beings we are imperfect; all of us make mistakes. The way we respond to these failings is what creates more, or lessens, stress in our lives. Our pattern of response is one we probably have been repeating since childhood. One way to change the pattern is through the use of verbal affirmations, positive statements that you repeat to yourself as often as possible during the day. Affirmations should be in the present tense, contain only positive words, and serve as a response to an often-heard negative message or as an expression of a goal.

For example, if some of the previous critical messages sound familiar to you, two affirmations that would help counteract them are: "I love and approve of myself" and "I am always doing the best I can." When people begin repeating affirmations, they usually don't believe what they're saying (that's why they're saying them), although they would like to. Using affirmations is like reprogramming a computer. Your subconscious mind is the computer that has been receiving the same message for years; now you are going to change the input.

Most computers have a total capacity for processing information far beyond the ability of the majority of computer operators to access it. Similarly, neuroscientists believe that the average person uses only 5 to 10 percent of his or her total brain capacity. This average person has about 50,000 thoughts every day, and it is estimated that 95 percent of them are the same ones he or she had the day before. Your brain hears the same "program" repeated over and over again. It's no wonder you are able to realize only a small fraction of your (and your brain's) full potential.

Mental health will help to develop your creativity—you'll be re-creating yourself—while allowing you greater access to the parts of your brain that have been dormant.

The best time to say your affirmation is immediately following the negative message you give yourself. I remember feeling so frustrated with my sinus headaches or congestion that I would think to myself, "This will never go away." After I began affirmations, I followed my hopeless comments with an immediate "My sinuses are now completely healed." This affirmation always made me feel a little better and gave me some hope. As my condition improved, I began to believe it more and more until it was actually true. Louise Hay has written a wonderful book on self-healing called *You Can Heal Your Life,* in which she focuses on the healing potential of affirmations as a means of learning to love yourself. Ms. Hay has a clinic in Santa Monica, California, for the treatment of AIDS. Her book contains a list of medical conditions, each with a corresponding affirmation. The one for sinusitis and bronchitis is "I declare peace and harmony are within me and surround me at all times; all is well." I used that one, too, to help cure my sinus disease. For allergies she suggests, "The world is safe and friendly. I am safe. I am at peace with life." For asthma, "It is safe now for me to take charge of my own life. I choose to be free." And for colds, "I allow my mind to relax and be at peace. Clarity and harmony are within me and around me."

You can use affirmations to help change any belief that doesn't feel good to you, or to help you achieve any goal. Most of my patients have come in because of one or more chronic physical or mental problems. Their objectives are clear: to stop having sinus infections or asthma attacks, to get rid of allergies, to stop living with chronic pain, to have more energy, to suffer less anxiety, and so forth. After they have begun to see a definite improvement in their physical condition, which is usually after they have been working on the physical and environmental aspects of the Sinus Survival Program for about one month, I recommend the following exercise:

- List your greatest talents and gifts. You have several. These are things that are most special about you, or that you do better than most other people. Ask yourself, "What do I most appreciate about myself?"
- Next, list the things you most enjoy—both activities and states of being, e.g., "I really enjoy just being in the mountains, or on a beach." There will be some overlap with your first list. Many of the activities you enjoy doing are the things you're best at.
- Now make a list of all your goals or objectives in every realm of your life—physical/environmental, mental, emotional, social, and spiritual. Physical and environmental goals can include recovering from illnesses or ailments, engaging in or mastering a particular physical activity (anything you've ever considered doing), or living or working in a certain place. Mental goals might address career plans, financial objectives, and any limiting beliefs that you'd like to change. Emotional goals have to do with feelings and self-esteem. Social goals are about your relationships with other people, while spiritual objectives have to do with your relationship with God or a power greater than yourself. As you do this part of the exercise, ask yourself, "What does my ideal life look like?" "Where do I see myself five or ten years from now?" "What is my purpose—what am I here to do?" Do *not* give yourself a time frame within which to attain any of these goals, and remember, it is *not* necessary to have a plan for getting there.
- Next, reword all of your goals into affirmations. For example, a goal might be "I'd like to cure my sinusitis." The affirmation could then be "My sinuses are now completely healed" or "My sinuses are getting better every day."
- Compile a list of affirmations that includes all of your goals, objectives, and any limiting beliefs that you'd like to change.
- Recite this entire list twice a day; and whenever you hear a negative, limiting, or critical message, recite the one affirmation that corresponds to that message. You can also choose to write them all down, reciting each one as you write, and then

visualize each one. Or you can record them onto a cassette and listen to them in your own voice. I've found that writing, reciting, and then visualizing your affirmations is the most effective method for manifesting your desires.

I learned this technique from a patient, a man who owns an oil company and works part-time as a psychotherapist. He had a terrible case of chronic sinusitis. On our second session, one month into the Sinus Survival Program, I presented this idea of changing some of his limiting, critical, or negative beliefs and clarifying his goals and objectives as a foundation of greater mental health. Shortly after this visit, he formulated a lengthy list of affirmations and goals. Once each day he recited every one of his new beliefs, then wrote them down on a sheet of paper, and after each one he closed his eyes and visualized what that desire or goal would look or feel like. When I next saw him, just over two months later, he told me that he had been repeating this procedure of reciting, writing, and visualizing for sixty consecutive days. He was thrilled to report to me that at least half of his affirmations and goals had already become a reality, including healthy sinuses! He continues to practice this method (using new affirmations) along with the physical and environmental health recommendations that he had implemented at the outset of the program. It is now more than two years since my third session with him. During that time he has had only one sinus infection, and his chronic sinusitis remains cured.

My patients' affirmation/goal lists provide a blueprint of our work together. The lists also become their personal vision and give direction to their own self-healing process.

You must be able to clarify your desires to have any chance of obtaining them, and as you do this exercise, try to be as specific as possible. The next step is to believe, however minimally, that it is possible for you to meet these goals. The more you repeat the affirmations, the stronger your belief will become.

The third step in this formula for self-realization is expectation. The stronger your belief and the more objectives you have already reached, the higher will be your level of expectation.

After my chronic sinusitis was cured, I developed the belief that anything is possible, one that has helped me to realize other dreams. Whatever it is that you *desire,* as long as you *believe* it's possible, you can *expect* it to happen. It is not necessary to know how, or to have a definite plan. Just be patient and flexible and be willing to accept the result even if the "package" in which it arrives is different from what you had envisioned. If your objectives are clear, your intuition will help you make the right decisions to get what you want. Remember that you can always choose what to believe. Rather than continuing with the attitude "I'll believe it when I see it," why not try "When I believe it, then I'll see it."

How you choose to see your sinus condition or any other chronic illness can play a vital role in the way the disease affects you and whether or not it goes away. Some of the early reactions to a chronic or life-threatening disease are denial ("There must be some mistake"), anger and frustration ("Why me?"; "What terrible luck"), self-pity ("I'll never be able to enjoy life again"), and resignation ("I'll just have to put up with it and continue to live this way for the rest of my life"). All of these are quite normal and understandable responses to something as devastating as a chronic illness. However, if you are interested in healing yourself, it is important to get beyond this point and look at your disease in a different light. According to Bernie Siegel, who contributed the following material to the book *Chop Wood, Carry Water,* you have several choices:

- Accept your illness. Being resigned to an illness can be destructive and can allow the illness to run your life, but accepting it allows energy to be freed for other things in your life.
- See the illness as a source of growth. If you begin to grow psychologically in response to the loss the illness has created in your life, then you don't need to have a physical illness anymore.
- View your illness as a positive redirection in your life. This means that you don't have to judge anything that

happens to you. If you get fired from a job, for example, assume that you are being redirected toward something else you are supposed to be doing. Your entire life changes when you say that something is just a redirection. You are then at peace. Everything is okay and you go on your way, knowing that the new direction is the one that is intrinsically right for you. After a while you begin to *feel* that this is true.

• Death or recurrence of illness is no longer seen as synonymous with failure after the aforementioned steps are accomplished, but simply as further choices or steps. If staying alive were your sole goal, you would have to be a failure because you do have to die someday. However, when you begin to accept the inevitability of death and see that you have only a limited time, you begin to realize that you might as well enjoy the present to the best of your ability.

• Learn self-love and peace of mind, and the body responds. Your body gets "live" or "energy" messages when you say "I love myself." That's not the ego talking, it's self-esteem. It's as if someone else is loving you, saying that you are a worthwhile person, believing in you, and telling you that you are here to give something to the world. When you do that, your immune system says, "This person likes living; let's fight for his or her life."

• Don't make physical change your sole goal. Seek peace of mind, acceptance, and forgiveness. Learn to love. In the process, the disease won't be totally overlooked—it will be seen as one of the problems you are having, and perhaps one of your fears. If you learn about hope, love, acceptance, forgiveness, and peace of mind, the disease might go away in the process.

• Achieve immortality through love. The only way you can live forever is to love somebody. Then you can really leave a gift behind. When you live that way, as many people with physical illnesses do, it is even possible to decide when you die. You can say, "Thank you, I've used my body to its limit. I have loved as much as I possibly can, and I'm leaving at two o'clock today." And you go. Then maybe you have spent half an hour dying and the rest of your life living; but when these things are not done, you might spend a lot of your life dying, and only a little living.

I realize that most of you do not have a terminal disease, just a case of good old chronic sinusitis or allergies, but each of these options for looking at physical illness can work for you as a form of preventive medicine. In my experience, chronic pain and imminent death have provided the greatest motivation for people to change, but why wait until you have reached that point of crisis?

A powerful technology for changing thoughts and beliefs is neurolinguistic programming (NLP). NLP teaches a wide variety of rapid and practical ways to change both feelings and beliefs through the use of goal setting, affirmations, and mental imagery. Developed in the early 1970s by information scientist Richard Bandler and linguistics professor John Grinder at the University of California, Santa Cruz, NLP offers a new perspective on how the mind works. It teaches us how to communicate with ourselves more powerfully by learning how to change the way we see ourselves, how we talk to ourselves, and how we feel about ourselves. It can be used as a method of therapy for eliminating unwanted responses and treating a variety of chronic ailments. It is also effective in transforming phobias and other traumatic responses; helping children and adults overcome learning disabilities; eliminating unwanted behaviors such as smoking, eating disorders, and insomnia; learning to excel in any area—sports, business, or school; and resolving conflicts between people and within yourself. NLP teaches the skills that promote positive change, which in turn can generate new possibilities and opportunities. You can learn more about NLP by reading about it in *Using Your Brain for a Change* by Richard Bandler, taking a class, or working with a certified NLP practitioner in your area.

WORK

Your job is another vital aspect of your mental health. Some questions you need to ask yourself are: "Do I enjoy my job?" "Does my work utilize my greatest talents?" "Is my job fulfilling and challenging?" I realize that for the majority of Americans the answer to these questions is no. Unfortunately, there is a significant physiological price to be paid for not loving your work. In a study on the risk factors for heart disease conducted in the late 1980s by the Massachusetts Department of Health, the two greatest risks lie in one's self-happiness rating and level of job satisfaction. Low scores on these two were shown to be better indicators of the likelihood for developing heart disease than high cholesterol, high blood pressure, overweight, and a sedentary lifestyle. The findings were further dramatized by the astounding statistic that more people died of heart attacks on Monday mornings around 9:00 than at any other time of the week! What a powerful demonstration of the mind-body connection.

Why, then, do so many of us continue to risk our lives and quality of life working in jobs that we dislike? The beliefs that are most often responsible are "I have no choice; I need the money"; "I'll never be able to make any money doing what I love to do"; or "I have no idea what I'd enjoy doing or what my greatest talents are." Every one of us has been blessed with at least one God-given gift. For most of us there is at least one activity that we enjoy doing or that we do quite well. *That* is where you begin to investigate what your gifts are.

Arnold Patent, in his book *You Can Have It All,* describes the universal principles that apply to obtaining one's life goals. He also suggests an exercise for identifying talents. It is as follows:

> Make a list of the things you love to do. Limit the list to those activities that create an excitement in you at the mere thought of them. The shorter the list, the easier it is

to reach the desired result. Select the item on the list that is most important to you. Do this no matter how much you may resist picking one item. Remember, picking one does not mean you have to give up the others forever. Make a list of the ways you can express the talent you just selected. It is best to do this daily. Keep a separate book for this exercise. Write down every idea that occurs to you, no matter how silly or meaningless it may seem. The purpose of the exercise is to stimulate your creative mind. After doing the exercise for a period of time, you will have developed a habit pattern that will continually produce creative ways to express what you love to do. The number of ways you can express yourself by doing what you love has no limit.

Scientists' belief that human beings make use of only a small fraction (about 5 to 10 percent) of their brain power lends credence to the statement that your capabilities are limitless. You need only acknowledge that you are seeking a greater level of fulfillment, are willing to change, are ready to take a risk (it could well be a greater risk not to), and will begin the exploration that will lead you to work that you love doing. What a wonderful treat to give to yourself!

MENTAL IMAGERY

This technique of visualization is one that each of us uses every day, but most of the time subconsciously. Our inner dialogue and the messages we continually give ourselves are very often accompanied by inner pictures. In a sense, these images are "waking dreams." Since the 1970s there has been a growing interest within the medical and other health professions in harnessing these images to be used as a conscious therapy. From the pioneering work of O. Carl Simonton, M.D., an oncologist working with cancer patients, to the experiences of ordinary physicians who have made mental imagery an integral part of their treatment, the results have been truly astounding. Even more exciting is the fact that the technique easily lends itself to self-healing, as long as you are willing to practice.

Martin Rossman, M.D., of the University of California Medical Center in San Francisco, and author of *Healing Yourself: A Step-by-Step Program for Better Health Through Imagery,* believes that imagery can lead to relief in 90 percent of the problems people bring to their primary care physician. From minor ailments such as back pain, neck pain, arthritis, palpitations, dizziness, and fatigue to conditions as serious as cancer and heart disease, patients can use imagery to address the mental and emotional aspects of their illnesses, thereby helping the physical healing.

I first became aware of mental imagery after hearing on a television talk show about a nine-year-old boy who had healed his inoperable cancerous brain tumor. He had spent about fifteen to twenty minutes daily sitting quietly with his eyes closed, while picturing missiles being fired into his tumor. The remission of his cancer was documented with brain scans. The description of this technique certainly captured my attention.

Shortly thereafter, I came down with yet another sinus infection. I decided to try mental imagery in addition to my usual regimen for the treatment of acute sinusitis. Without having received any formal training in the method, I sat in a straight-backed chair and focused on deep, relaxed breathing for about twenty minutes. The following vision appeared to me. I saw a large sphere completely covered with a slimy, moldy, greenish-gray crud—terrible-looking stuff! At the top of this globe (if you picture the earth, this would be the North Pole) were a group of ten little workmen, clothed in overalls and caps, each holding a high-powered hose and a long-handled push broom. I watched as they methodically began to work their way down the sides of this sphere, hosing and sweeping away the green slime. Underneath was revealed the brightest and healthiest-looking orange I had ever seen. After the orange was completely uncovered, I got up from my chair and at that moment felt the largest clump of postnasal mucus I'd ever had in the back of my throat. As I marveled at the size of the greenish-yellow mass I had then spit into the sink, I could sense that my sinus infection was almost completely resolved. It never returned. Needless to say, I remain impressed with the power of mental imagery to treat physical ailments, although it is not the only therapy I used to cure my sinus disease. Another image you can use preventively for sinuses is to begin each day seeing yourself surrounded by several layers of bright, multicolored light. This light can act as a protective shield or as your own personal air filter removing air pollutants before they can enter your nose and sinuses. A very handy image indeed, especially in badly polluted environments.

An effective image for asthma or bronchitis might be one in which you visualize your lungs being light, unrestricted, free to inflate like a blown-up balloon; and the airways being wide open, "Roto-Rooted," washed clean of the thick mucus; or a "magic" solution being flushed into them that dissolves all of the mucus and heals the scarred and inflamed tissue as it rushes through the tubes restoring the mucous membrane to its normal pink robust condition. It need not be anatomically correct, just a vision that represents your body's physical dysfunction and some action that corrects it.

Take only five or ten minutes a day to sit comfortably with your eyes closed in a quiet place; focus on your breath, and see what your mind conjures up for you. It is a totally effortless yet powerful and energizing technique requiring little or no training, and just a little bit of your time.

Mental imagery can also be employed to help you feel more relaxed and peaceful, develop your creative talents, create more fulfillment in relationships, reach your career goals (the clarity of a goal is definitely enhanced when you picture it on a regular basis), and dissolve negative habit patterns. To learn more about this technique, I recommend Dr. Rossman's book; *Healing Visualizations: Creating Health Through Imagery* by Gerald Epstein, M.D., a professor of psychiatry at Mt. Sinai Medical Center in

New York; and *Creative Visualization* by Shakti Gawain, an extraordinary teacher of holistic health.

OPTIMISM AND HUMOR

It may come as a surprise to learn that an optimistic outlook and a good, hearty laugh are beneficial not only mentally but physically. In the research for their book *Healthy Pleasures,* Robert Ornstein, Ph.D., and David Sobel, M.D., found that the healthiest people are optimistic and happy and seem to feel that things will work out no matter what their difficulties. As Ornstein and Sobel put it, "The way they live and envision their lives nourishes their life itself. They expect good things of the world. They expect that their world will be orderly; they expect that other people will like and respect them; and most important, they expect pleasure in much of what they do."

Many of these people maintain a vital sense of humor about life and enjoy a good laugh, more often than not at their own expense. Studies have shown that laughter can improve the function of the immune system. Hearty laughter can be considered a gentle exercise of the body, a form of "inner jogging." Ornstein and Sobel describe the physical effects of laughter:

> A robust laugh gives the muscles of your face, shoulders, diaphragm, and abdomen a good workout. With convulsive or side-splitting laughter, even your arm and leg muscles come into play. Your heart rate and blood pressure temporarily rise, breathing becomes faster and deeper, and oxygen surges through your bloodstream. A vigorous laugh can burn up as many calories per hour as brisk walking or cycling. . . . The afterglow of a hearty laugh is positively relaxing. Blood pressure may temporarily fall, your muscles go limp, and you bask in a mellow euphoria. Some researchers speculate that laughter triggers the release of endorphins, the brain's own opiates; this may ac-

count for the pain relief and euphoria that accompany laughter.

Some believe that it is possible to treat disease through laughter. The Gesundheit Institute in Arlington, Virginia, founded and directed by Patch Adams, M.D., focuses on the healing potential of humor. Norman Cousins, in his best-seller *Anatomy of an Illness,* attributed his recovery from ankylosing spondylitis (a potentially crippling arthritic condition) to the many hours he spent watching Marx Brothers movies and reruns of the television show "Candid Camera."

There is some evidence that laughter strengthens the immune system. In one study, research subjects watching a videotape of the comedian Richard Pryor temporarily produced in their saliva elevated levels of antibodies that help combat infections such as colds. Interestingly, the subjects who said they frequently used humor to cope with life stress had consistently higher baseline levels of those protective antibodies.

As Ornstein and Sobel express it, "Laughter is an affirmation of our humanness and an effective antidote to adversity. It can free us to detach and consider problems along new, creative lines. Laughter is a celebration of the unconventional, the unusual, the irregular, the indecorous, the illogical, the nonsensical." The only side effect to this powerful medicine is pleasure. When the question posed to octogenarians is "If you had your life to live over again, what would you do differently?" the answer often is "I'd take life much less seriously." Comedian George Burns, at ninety-five years of age, wrote the book *Wisdom of the 90s.* He attributes his ability to laugh at himself as well as loving what he does for a living as the most important factors in his longevity.

If you are interested in learning a more pleasurable approach to the entire spectrum of holistic health, *Healthy Pleasures* is an excellent resource.

FORGIVENESS

There might not be a concept more important to mental fitness than that of forgiveness. How often have you thought to yourself, "I am my own worst enemy," or "I sure do make things hard on myself"? Or do you often find yourself blaming someone else for your own problems or stress? The next time you are aware of blaming others, physically point your index finger at them (or preferably their images) and take a look at where the other three curled fingers of that hand are pointed. Forgiveness begins with accepting responsibility for the role you play in shaping your life's experiences. You cannot practice forgiveness on anyone else before starting on yourself. The affirmations "I am always doing the best I can" and "I acknowledge and accept that I am the creative power in my world" are both helpful in learning to forgive yourself. The latter affirmation also happens to be Louise Hay's recommendation for postnasal drip.

Stephen Levine, in his book *Healing into Life and Death,* devotes an excellent chapter to forgiveness. It begins with the following sentence: "The beginning of the path of healing is the end of life unlived." It also contains a forgiveness meditation that I often recommend to my patients.

Albert Ellis, Ph.D., a psychologist and founder of the Institute for Rational-Emotive Therapy in New York City, has probably done more psychotherapy sessions than any other psychologist: some 90,000 hours' worth. The following quote of his, from an article by Claire Warga titled "You Are What You Think" in *Psychology Today* (September 1988), helped me better understand the importance of forgiveness in the spectrum of mental health. Ellis said, "My psychotherapeutic philosophy holds that the vast majority of humans, in every part of the world, are much more disturbed than they have to be because they simply will not accept themselves as fallible, incessantly error-prone humans."

You can learn a great deal about forgiveness by watching or (preferably) playing sports. Imagine, for example, a tennis player in an important match. Suppose he misses a shot he thinks he should have made. His response can run the gamut from mild disappointment, as evidenced by a facial expression, to obvious rage, with loud self-berating and racket-throwing. In order to continue to play at an optimal level of performance and remain competitive, he must be able to very quickly forgive himself for having made this bad shot (mistake), since he will have to attempt many more shots in rapid succession. If he continues to hold onto his anger or his belief that he's a bad player for having made a mistake, he will soon lose his confidence, his ability to concentrate, and the match.

This same type of scenario occurs for most of us on a daily basis, although usually not in the sports arena. Although we might have more time than the tennis player to recover from our mistakes, unless we forgive ourselves and let go of the past, we will lose some degree of confidence, the ability to focus and stay in the present, and the capacity to do as well as we know we are capable of doing.

How, then, does the commonly held belief "I know I did not do as well as I am capable of doing" correlate with the affirmation "I am always doing the best I can"? Given all of the circumstances of your life—where and how you were raised, your level of education and training, and the present conditions of your personal life and current level of stress—at every moment of every day, you and I and everyone else are always doing the best we can. That is my belief. To me it feels much better than the alternative, and as you practice it on yourself you will be forgiving others at the same time.

For many high achievers, a capacity for forgiveness has been a critical factor in their success. In order to grow, learn, expand your horizons, and find greater fulfillment in life, you must be willing to change, take risks, and try something new. This cannot be done without making "mistakes," which can also be looked upon as opportunities to learn (just as Bernie Siegel felt illness could be seen as a source of growth). By taking risks you provide yourself an excellent opportunity to practice self-forgiveness. As with anything else, the more you practice, the better you become. "I am always doing the best I can" is not a belief that precludes trying to do better. It allows you the chance to do just that, by helping you to stay in the game, without destroying your self-confidence. It also makes risk-taking and life in general much more fun. If it feels right to you, why not choose this belief? While you're at it, you can add the corollary, "There are no mistakes; only lessons."

MENTAL HEALTH RECOMMENDATIONS: A SUMMARY

Beliefs and affirmations: Identify negative beliefs you would like to change and put your responses into the form of affirmations. Some that are almost always helpful are the following:

I am always doing the best I can.
I love and approve of myself.
I love my body.
Everything is happening at just the right time.
My _____ (sinuses, nose, lungs, etc.) are getting better every day.

For chronic sinusitis and bronchitis, add the following:

I declare peace and harmony are within me and surround me at all times.

For allergies:

The world is safe and friendly. I am safe. I am at peace with life.
I am comfortable in any environment.

For asthma:

It is safe now for me to take charge of my own life. I choose to be free.
I am always breathing freely and deeply.

- *Goals:* Make a list of your goals, desires, and objectives in every realm of holistic health (physical, environmental, mental, emotional, spiritual, and social), as long as you believe that they are even remotely possible. Put them into the form of affirmations and add them to your other affirmations to form a composite list. Repeat these regularly either orally or in writing, or both; or record them on a cassette and play them back daily. Listening is not as effective as speaking, writing, and visualizing. Doing these three together is best.

- *Choice:* Recognize that you are a unique individual and can choose your own beliefs based on your intuition or whatever feels right for you. Choose to accept your chronic illness as an opportunity for psychological growth, redirection, and ultimately greater enjoyment of your life.

- Desire, belief, and expectation: These will help you achieve any goal. Optimism (the expectation that things will work out well) is also an ingredient found in most healthy people.

- *NLP:* This helps to change beliefs and attitudes, and is a method for excelling in any endeavor (e.g., business, sports, or the creative or performing arts). It should be learned from a certified NLP practitioner. To excel in anything can improve your self-esteem.

- *Work:* Find a job that you love doing and that employs your unique talents. Avoid work environments with especially unhealthy air. Do the Arnold Patent exercise described in this chapter.

- *Humor:* Look for more humor and opportunities for laughter in your life. Lighten up; take life less seriously.

- *Forgiveness:* Remember that you are a human being with imperfections, weaknesses, and flaws, as is everyone else. Learn to accept your mistakes and avoid blaming others. Affirmations can help with this.

Chapter 11

EMOTIONAL HEALTH

The emotionally fit are able to identify their feelings and can express, fully experience, and accept them as well. I have heard contemporary American culture referred to as the "no-feeling" society. The feelings are certainly present, but as a result of our lifestyle we have constructed such formidable protective barriers around ourselves that to a great extent we have become unconscious of our feelings, especially the more uncomfortable ones.

There are those who believe there are only two basic human emotions: love and fear. The so-called negative or painful emotions, such as anger, anxiety, depression, envy, guilt, hatred, hostility, jealousy, loneliness, shame, and worry, are all expressions of fear. The feelings of acceptance, intimacy, joy, power, and peacefulness are all aspects of love. The greater our degree of fear, the less capable we are of experiencing love.

There are other mental health professionals who consider four basic emotions: love or joy, sadness, anger, and fear. So at any given moment, you're feeling either glad, sad, mad, or scared, or some combination of these. In our culture it is not socially acceptable to express most of the "negative" emotions, and men especially are not supposed to show signs of weakness or insecurity or to cry ("Big boys don't cry"). The majority of us have learned to repress these feelings until we are unaware that we even have them. Society has helped us suppress our painful (negative) feelings by perpetuating the myth of an emotionally pain-free existence. The numerous ads in the media for analgesics to treat tension headaches and the common use of alcohol or drugs to dull the pain of an awkward social situation or personal crisis give us the relentless message that not only is *pain a bad thing,* but life can be pain free.

If we spent less time avoiding emotional pain, but instead focused our attention on it, accepted it, and relaxed into it, the pain would diminish or even disappear. If we continue to ignore and repress it, it often manifests itself as physical pain, illness, or disease. Redford Williams, M.D., a researcher in behavioral medicine at the Duke University Medical Center, has gathered a wealth of data suggesting that chronic anger is so damaging to the body that it ranks with, or even exceeds, cigarette smoking, obesity, and a high-fat diet as a powerful risk factor for early death. Williams reported that people who scored high on a hostility scale as teenagers were much more likely than their more cheerful peers to have elevated cholesterol levels as adults, suggesting a link between unremitting anger and heart disease.

In another recent study, Dr. Mara Julius, an epidemiologist at the University of Michigan, analyzed the effects of chronic anger on women over a period of eighteen years. She found that women who had answered initial test questions with obvious signs of long-term, suppressed anger were three times more likely to have died during the study than those women who did not harbor such hostile feelings. In fact, chronic sinusitis is usually associated with a tremendous amount of unexpressed anger.

Clyde Reid is director of the Center for New Beginnings in Denver. In his insightful book *Celebrate the Temporary,* he says, "Leaning into life's pain can also be a lifestyle, and is far more satisfying than the avoidance style. It requires small doses of plain courage to look pain in the eye, but it prepares you for more serious pain when it comes. In the meantime, all the energy expended to avoid pain is now available for the business of living."

I am not advocating that you seek out painful experiences, nor am I proposing that you endure prolonged or persistent pain. That is called suffering. Health and happiness do not have prerequisites that require you to suffer. Life is to be enjoyed, but the notion that it can be lived entirely without painful feelings is an unhealthy belief. Pain and joy are intertwined, and the more you allow yourself to accept, embrace, and feel pain, the greater will be your sense of emotional health.

MENTAL/EMOTIONAL OVERLAP

Although mental health focuses primarily on thoughts, beliefs, attitudes, and imagery, and emotional health on feelings, they are for the most part inextricably related. Together they comprise the "mind" aspect of holistic health—body, mind, and spirit. Although I consider social and spiritual health to be components of "spirit," all four are so interrelated that improvement in one area will often have positive ramifications in the others. I have dealt with them separately to enable you to better grasp the scope of each aspect of health and to make it easier to work on each one.

Of the mental-emotional connection, Albert Ellis has said that "virtually all 'emotionally disturbed' individuals actually think crookedly, magically, dogmatically, and unrealistically." David D. Burns, M.D., is the director of the Behavioral Science Research Foundation and acting chairman of psychiatry at the Presbyterian Medical Center of Philadelphia. In *The Feeling Good Handbook: Using the New Mood Therapy in Everyday Life,* he writes:

> Certain kinds of negative thoughts make people unhappy. In fact, I believe that unhealthy, negative emotions—depression, anxiety, excessive anger, inappropriate guilt, etc. —are *always* caused by illogical, distorted thoughts, even if those thoughts may seem absolutely valid at the time. By learning to look at things more realistically, by getting rid of your distorted thinking patterns, you can break out of a

bad mood, often in a short period of time, without having to rely on medication or prolonged psychotherapy.

Burns offers the following list of thought distortions:

- All-or-nothing thinking. You classify things into absolute, black-and-white categories.
- Overgeneralization. You view a single negative situation as a never-ending pattern of defeat.
- Mental filtering. You dwell on negatives and overlook positives.
- Discounting the positive. You insist your accomplishments or positive qualities "don't count."
- Magnification or minimization. You blow things out of proportion or shrink their importance inappropriately.
- Making "should" statements. You criticize yourself and others by using the terms *should, shouldn't, must, ought,* and *have to.*
- Emotional reasoning. You reason from how you feel. If you feel like an idiot, you assume you must be one. If you don't feel like doing something, you put it off.
- Jumping to conclusions. You "mind read," assuming, without definite evidence of it, that people are reacting negatively to you. Or you "fortune tell," arbitrarily predicting bad outcomes.
- Labeling. You identify with your shortcomings. Instead of saying, "I made a mistake," you tell yourself, "I'm such a jerk . . . a real loser."
- Personalization and blame. You blame yourself for something you weren't entirely responsible for, or you blame others and ignore the impact of your own attitudes or behavior.

It is now widely accepted that negative thoughts and the feelings they engender contribute to physical illness. Conversely, recent research has revealed that positive emotions cause the body to produce substances that are identical to the ingredients in pharmaceutical drugs that help people feel better. For example, when you feel peace and tranquility, your body makes molecules identical to those in the tranquilizer Valium. When you feel exhilarated, your body produces interleuken-2—in its pharmaceutical form, a powerful anticancer drug, each dose of which costs nearly $40,000. If you were to engage in an especially fun-filled activity, your body might make millions of dollars' worth of interleuken-2.

PSYCHOTHERAPY

Traditional psychotherapy based on Freudian principles has been the conventional approach to the treatment of mental and emotional disorders. Like traditional medicine, this is a disease-oriented approach, in which patients come to be fixed. Still, psychiatrists, psychoanalysts, and psychotherapists might have distinctly different ways of treating the same problem.

Today, the majority of patients who see psychiatrists are labeled with a psychiatric diagnosis and treated with psychotherapeutic drugs. The arsenal of these drugs is constantly expanding as researchers explore the physiology of the human brain. In fact, Prozac, one of the newer antidepressants, has quickly risen almost to the top of the list of most prescribed drugs in this country. Psychiatry is definitely moving in the direction of less counseling and more drug therapy, although every one of these drugs has potentially unpleasant side effects. The emphasis is on treating the symptom with drugs rather than encouraging the patient to change attitudes or behavior, or just to be with their pain and learn from it.

A new wrinkle in psychotherapy is the rapidly expanding field of cognitive therapy. Therapist and theorist Albert Ellis has pioneered a psychotherapy that stresses the importance of cognitions —ideas, beliefs, assumptions, interpretations, and thinking processes—in the origins and treatment of emotional disturbance. There are many different types of cognitive therapies, all of which teach people how to evaluate critically their own thought processes and to trust in their own reasoning ability, rather than adhere to the standards and norms of others. These theories are based on the power of people to transform their current beliefs. Unlike the Freudian approach, the focus is not on the past but on the present: *If you can change what you think, you'll change the way you feel.* In a society that looks for fast solutions, this brief form of psychotherapy usually takes under a year, much less time than the traditional psychotherapeutic approach.

Increasingly, the job of counseling is being assumed by psychologists, social workers, pastoral counselors, and anyone else with a counseling degree. The health care industry, particularly the medical insurance companies, has helped to create these changes. It has discouraged long-term psychotherapy by reimbursing for a limited number of visits to the therapist; by paying for only a portion of the fee, with a large copayment assumed by the patient; or by not paying for this service at all.

Although this book is intended to be a self-help guide, and holistic medicine focuses on self-healing, I strongly advocate psychotherapy as an important means of improving your health. In addition to the obvious mental and emotional benefits, physical effects have now also been documented. Norman Cousins conducted a study at the UCLA School of Medicine that involved two groups of cancer patients. The group that had psychotherapy for one and a half hours a week for six weeks showed profound positive changes in their immune systems. The group that received no counseling had no change in immune function.

More and more therapists are becoming aware of the connection between psychotherapy and spiritual growth, and have incorporated spirituality into their therapeutic program. I encourage you to seek a therapist who has made this transition and who understands and appreciates the importance of spirituality in the healing process. I would also recommend someone who practices cognitive therapy. The therapist should be someone with whom you feel comfortable. It would be prudent to interview several before selecting one.

Goals are extremely important. Try to clarify what it is you want from psychotherapy. Be as specific as possible. The greater your clarity, the shorter your therapy. However, you might be in such emotional pain that drug therapy sounds very good to you, and that might be just what you need. Find a psychiatrist and get started. You also have the option of seeing a holistic physician. It should be apparent from this text that psychotherapy is one aspect of such a physician's job.

There are times when the symptoms of disease—whether physical or mental—can be so overwhelming that people feel paralyzed or suicidal. Life seems to be at a standstill and they feel worthless and are without hope. You must determine your own threshold of discomfort. When it has been reached, seek help in a way that feels best to you. This is your program, and no one knows you better than you do. To achieve a balanced state of holistic health, you cannot allow yourself to get stuck in one area for too long. Try to learn something from each experience, and then move on. In some instances, this can take a year or more. Whether you are suffering from the death of a loved one, a divorce, a business failure, or a chronic or terminal disease, you must go through a period of grieving and adjust to your loss. Elisabeth Kübler-Ross, M.D., a psychiatrist and author of the classic text *On Death and Dying,* has identified five stages in this process: denial, anger, bargaining, depression, and then acceptance. Allow yourself to feel all of your feelings, and know that there is something to be gained from them. Realize that however miserable you feel, it is only temporary. Remember that to live without pain is to live an incomplete life.

MEDITATION AND BREATHING THERAPY

As a society, I believe we do not allow ourselves to feel, but how do we manage to avoid our feelings? Workaholism might be the most common means of escape. Our minds are so busy with important thoughts that there is neither room nor time for feelings. Another means of escape, drug abuse, has become such a threat to our culture's stability that our government declared a war on drugs. That's fine, but it is only another example of symptomatic treatment. With all the publicity and billions of dollars that were spent on this campaign, I never heard any drug enforcement official question why so many millions of people have risked their lives to avoid confronting their feelings. Our extremely fast-paced society and its quick-fix syndrome are other symptoms of avoidance; we are eager for fast and easy ways to satisfy our needs for food, sex, money, energy, entertainment, exercise, transportation, communication, and health.

Why the hurry? Where are we running? The quest for money, power, material wealth, recognition, and intellectual superiority have become major distractions and, in many instances, addictions. Life could be infinitely more enjoyable and enriching if we would just slow down! We can smell the roses or simply tune in to life—to the messages our bodies are always giving us, to what we are thinking and feeling, to the value of our relationships, and to our connection to the earth and to our fellow human beings.

One way to slow down is to learn to breathe more consciously. For most of us, breathing is an unconscious process that begins traumatically at birth. After that, little attention is paid to breathing other than the ability to keep on doing it. The medical profession has not been curious as to how humans can improve this unconscious function by doing it more efficiently and consciously.

Meditation is one of several disciplines that can be described as conscious breathing. Meditation has several benefits. It slows you down and allows you to inhale more oxygen, which is, after all, the most critical nutrient for human health. Meditation is relaxing (it is an integral part of most stress management programs) and keeps you focused on the present, not allowing you to hang onto past regrets or worries about the future. It can empty your mind of thoughts and, if practiced enough, can help to bring more feelings to the surface, allow creative ideas to flow, and heighten spiritual awareness. It is also quite effective in lowering high blood pressure, slowing the heart rate, reducing pain (especially headaches), and is an adjunct in treating heart disease and many other physical ailments. Former Harvard researcher

Charles Alexander, Ph.D., taught transcendental meditation to a group of nursing-home patients. In 1990, he reported that over a three-year period, all the meditators survived, compared with only 62.6 percent of the nonmeditators.

Ideally, meditation should be practiced in a quiet place. Sit on the floor cross-legged or in a chair with your feet on the floor and your back unsupported. Abdominal breathing should be done through your nose at a rate of approximately three full breaths (inhale and exhale) per minute. To practice, place a hand on your belly: In abdominal breathing, your abdomen will protrude with each inhalation and flatten with each exhalation. To stay focused on the breath and avoid being distracted by your thoughts (they will be there, but just let them come and go), it helps to repeat silently a very short affirmation or just one word, such as *love, peace,* or whatever you'd like, on both inhalation and exhalation. At first try doing it for five minutes a day, then gradually increase the time to twenty minutes twice a day. Another technique you could try is to count slowly and silently to five ("one thousand one, one thousand two," etc.) on the inhalation, hold your breath for a count of five, exhale for five, then pause for five before beginning the next cycle. Don't be discouraged if this feels difficult at first. Sitting and breathing without thinking, listening to music, or obviously accomplishing something is not easy for most Americans. I can assure you, though, that if you continue to practice, you will soon begin to appreciate the many benefits of this simple routine. The next time you feel especially stressed, pay attention to the way you are breathing. You will probably find that your breaths are shallow and irregular; many people even hold their breath when they're anxious. This would be an ideal time to give a five-minute meditation a try. Meditation can also be a good way to start the day (it's energizing in the morning) and as a means of unwinding after work or before bed (it's relaxing later in the day). Books on meditation are widely available. I would recommend the following: *Wherever You Go, There You Are: Mindfulness Meditation in Everyday Life,* by Jon Kabat-Zinn, Ph.D.; *Concentration,* by Ernest Wood; and *A Gradual Awakening,* by Stephen Levine.

Yoga is another discipline of conscious breathing combined with movement. One of the asanas (yogic exercises), called the lion, is especially effective in helping the sinuses to drain. It relaxes facial muscles and in so doing, the ostia open and sinus pressure can be relieved. According to Mardi Erdmann, a former noted yoga instructor and author of *Undercover Exercise,* the lion is performed in the following manner: sit with your hands (palms down) on your thighs and your eyes closed; take a deep breath through your nose, your face quiet and relaxed but poised for action. On the exhale, open your eyes and mouth wide, stick your tongue way out (down to your chin), extend your hands and arms straight out in front of you with your fingers extended wide; your breath is forced out of your mouth over the tongue with an accompanying air sound (*not* a voice sound). I have previously mentioned the value of yoga as part of the holistic treatment program for asthma.

There are many varieties of breath therapy, sometimes referred to as "breath work." What they have in common is the ability to make you more aware of deeply held and often painful feelings. Breath therapies are similar to meditation in that they use the focus on breath to empty the mind of thoughts, but they differ in the style of breathing. Most breath therapies use the technique of connected breathing, which is much more rapid than the breathing of meditation. Each inhalation immediately follows the exhalation of the preceding breath. Mouth breathing is usually recommended, and both abdominal and chest breathing are used. The therapy can be performed even more effectively under water with the use of a snorkel. Two of the more popular breath therapies are rebirthing and holotropic therapy, in which loud music accompanies the breathing. I would suggest attempting breath work only under the direction of a skilled breath therapist. Because of the emotional release that results from this work, these experts often include psychotherapy as a part of the process. The therapist I have worked with is supervised by a psychiatrist. Although the field is still in its infancy, breath therapy is being recognized as a powerful tool for emotional health.

DREAMS AND JOURNALING

"Dreams are extraordinarily reliable commentaries on the life you really live—the people you care about, the events you anticipate, the problems you are trying to solve," says Robert Langs, M.D., a psychoanalyst and chief of the Center for Communicative Research at Beth Israel Hospital in New York City. "Every dream reflects an unconscious response to an emotionally charged situation in waking reality. [Dreams] consistently point out aspects of your feelings that you have overlooked, ignored, or tried to keep at bay. My own studies have indicated that the very process of remembering a dream promotes emotional stability. Analyzing dreams is an extremely helpful way of maintaining your equilibrium and your emotional balance."

There are at least two obstacles that prevent us from using our dreams as tools for better emotional health. First, most dreams are quickly forgotten. Second, the few that we do remember are filled with symbolism and imagery that do not lend themselves to simple interpretation. Dr. Langs believes that it is more natural to forget a dream than to remember it, because of our unconscious efforts to protect ourselves from mental and emotional pain. He thinks that we should trust our unconscious intuition. "When the conscious mind is ready to cope with the meanings embedded in a dream," he says, "in most instances you will dream some other version of it later—and remember it."

If you are able to recall dreams and would like to use them in your self-healing process, keep a pad and pencil or a tape recorder by your bed. By writing dreams down or verbally recording them immediately after you awaken, you will retain more of the details. The more often you do this, the better you may be able to understand the symbolism of your dreams. There are psychotherapists, usually with a Jungian orientation, who are skilled in dream interpretation and can help you. Three books I recommend are: *Do You Dream?* by Tony Crisp, which offers many alternative interpretations of symbols; *The Dictionary of*

Symbols by J. E. Cirlot; and *What Your Dreams Teach You* by Alex Lukeman. A dream, however, is highly personal and, ultimately, the dreamer is the only one who can appreciate its deepest meanings.

Journaling is the keeping of a written record of your feelings, thoughts, and any other information you'd like to clarify for yourself. If journaling is done on a regular basis it can increase self-knowledge and be both enlightening and enlivening. In a sense you become your own therapist or your own best friend; instead of trying to convey what you're feeling to another person, you're telling it to yourself. Communicating with yourself this way seems to allow for greater clarity and ease, probably because there is much less concern about judgment—you are the only one who will be reading what you write, and you don't have to worry about spelling or grammar. In the book *Opening Up,* James W. Pennebaker, Ph.D., documents the benefits to one's physical health that can be gained by writing about upsetting or traumatic experiences. If you write on a regular basis, your journal becomes an emotional "diary."

EMOTIONAL RELEASE

The two most recognized emotional ailments are anxiety and depression. I have found anger to be a component of both, but especially the latter. In fact, many psychiatrists believe that repressed anger is the "fuel" for depression. Although it is not always apparent to my patients, it has become clear to me that anger is almost universally present both as a cause and as a feeling that helps to maintain chronic sinusitis.

Anger is a perfectly normal human emotion. We usually feel some degree of anger on a daily basis. But anger has been stigmatized, and its expression is usually unacceptable. Much of the negative attitude toward anger has to do with fears about how this strong feeling will affect or be perceived by others. We're often afraid that our anger will hurt someone else, or that we may be perceived as harsh, abrasive, offensive, cruel, or even emotionally unstable. Comments such as "He's in a rage," "She really flew off the handle," or "Don't go near him, he's having a fit" help to reinforce our fear of expressing anger. Much of the time we repress it so quickly and unconsciously that we may not even know that we are mad. I have seen many patients who have had this conditioned response since early childhood, and are so adept that they are unaware of what they have been doing.

The medical profession has endorsed psychotherapy as the best means to deal with "excessive" anger and fear (i.e., depression and anxiety, along with a host of other emotional disorders). The traditional vehicles for treating these conditions are drug therapy and counseling. Both are mental or mind-focused tools. Drugs affect the brain directly, and most psychotherapy is a verbal and intellectual exercise that may take years to complete.

In recent years some psychotherapists have begun teaching their clients methods of using sound or their own bodies to quickly and effectively release anger. Not surprisingly, the most common of these techniques is screaming. It certainly worked well when we were young kids. The most difficult problem with screaming is finding a place where you won't attract attention or be considered crazy. Doing it in the basement of your home, in a closet, or in the car with the windows rolled up are all possibilities. If you want to make less noise you can hold your hands over your mouth when you scream. Take a deep abdominal breath just before screaming, and try to bring up the sound from your diaphragm or deep in your chest, and not from your throat, in order to protect your vocal cords. Slowly move your upper body or trunk from side to side and up and down while you're screaming (this will be a real challenge if you're sitting in your car). Two or three screams in succession are enough.

Punching is another effective method for venting anger. I have a heavy punching bag and boxing gloves, and I make daily visits to the basement for just a couple of minutes of punching. I do this preventively rather than waiting until I'm in a rage. However, when I do feel a lot of anger, punching is a great way to release it. Instead of a punching bag, you can also hit or punch pillows or your sofa, using your fists or a baseball bat or broomstick.

If you have young children, the Yogi Bear Bop Bag may help you teach the same technique. A gift of this toy shows that you accept and approve of your children's anger. You can encourage them to pretend that the Bop Bag is either you or their brother or sister or whomever it is they are angry at. A friend of mine has done this with his children and it works quite well. What a gift of emotional health to give your kids—to let them know that it's okay to be angry and to provide them with an acceptable means of expressing it.

Another technique involves stamping the floor with your right foot (first raise your knee waist high) while simultaneously bringing your right arm across your chest, elbow bent, and then forcefully bringing it back to its original position just as your foot hits the floor. This movement is accompanied by a grunt. Then repeat the same thing on the left side. Continue alternating sides for three to four minutes. When you've finished you'll feel a bit tired but much more relaxed.

I had one patient who interrupted as I began explaining anger release and said, "I don't have a problem with that. I go to a discount store and buy some cheap glasses, and whenever I get really angry I throw them against a brick wall and feel much better."

If none of these physical methods interests you, then try talking to yourself or expressing your anger to your spouse, another family member, close friend, or directly to the person with whom you are angry. Whatever feels comfortable to you is fine, but choose *something* and try it. Anger release has been extremely helpful for sinus sufferers.

Screaming is not the only method of emotional release left behind in early childhood. For men especially, crying is a luxury that is seldom indulged. In our society men cry only one-fifth as often as women do. Somewhere are "oceans" of tears that Americans have not allowed themselves to shed. Yet recent evidence from tear researcher William Frey suggests that the tears produced by emotional crying, as opposed to those triggered by injury or physical pain, may help the body release stress and dispose of toxic substances. Tears also contain endorphins, the adrenal hormone ACTH, the ovarian hormone prolactin (in women's tears only), and growth hormones, all of which are released by stress.

The vast majority of people report that crying improves mood and offers a welcome release of tensions. Interestingly enough, a recent study revealed that the majority of women release their anger through tears. At least one study of men and women with peptic ulcers or colitis showed that they were less likely to cry compared to their healthy peers. These patients were more likely to regard crying as a sign of weakness or loss of control. It may not be easy at first, but if you feel the tears coming, let go and allow them to flow. Crying is a healthy thing to do, both physically and emotionally.

I learned another emotional quick fix from the book *The Performance Edge,* by Robert K. Cooper, Ph.D. He calls it the Instant Calming Sequence (ICS), and it takes just thirty seconds to do and can be learned quickly and used effectively to relieve stress.

- Step 1: Breathe Easy
Surprisingly, most of us halt our breathing for several seconds or more at the first sign of stress. That reduces oxygen to the brain and increases feelings of anxiety. The ICS approach is simple: focus on continuing to breathe—smoothly, deeply, evenly—when pressure hits.
- Step 2: Flash a Smile
Learn to relax your face into a little smile—or at least don't frown—when you find yourself in a tight spot. Stress researchers say that the slightest smile—even when you don't feel like smiling—may increase blood flow to the brain and help "reset" the nervous system so it's less reactive to stress.
- Step 3: Shift Your Stance
A common stress response, known as somatic retraction, is

to assume a slouching posture: chest tightened or collapsed, shoulders rolled forward and down, abdomen, back, or neck tensed. This position not only restricts breathing and blood flow to the brain, it also creates muscle tension, slows reaction time, and can magnify any feelings of panic. The solution: just shift your body around. Pretend a skyhook is gently lifting your spinal column upward from a point on the top of your head. You'll feel less tense when your head is up, neck long, shoulders broad and loose, pelvis and hips level, back straight, and abdomen tension free. Also, simply changing positions—getting up if you're sitting, sitting down if you're standing —can do a lot to release pent-up emotions.

• Step 4: Do a Tension Check

Another common stress reaction is to unconsciously tighten muscles in the jaw, neck, back, shoulders, and/or abdomen. To release the tension, first locate your knots and tight spots by taking a fast mental scan of all your muscles, from clenched jaws to curled toes. Just doing this should signal your body to relax.

• Step 5: Pause, Then React

In the critical first instant of a challenge, you're better off pausing for a moment to acknowledge reality, clear your mind, and focus on the situation—then make a quick, appropriate response. Don't think that a momentary pause will make you appear weak or indecisive. On the contrary, by heading off counterproductive responses, such as anger, or victimizing thoughts, it helps you regain your powers of alertness and concentration, and get back in control.

PLAY

Play is another thing that many of us have relegated to childhood. As a means of expressing joy, passion, exhilaration, and at times even ecstasy, play is an essential component of emotional health. The word itself comes from the Dutch *pleien,* meaning "to dance, leap for joy, and rejoice." The notion that play is something to be abandoned as soon as you grow up and get a job is an unhealthy belief. In fact, if you've found a job that you love doing, then work and play can become almost indistinguishable. As George Halas, former owner of the Chicago Bears football team, once said, "It's only work if there's someplace else you'd rather be." If your work encompasses your greatest talents or gifts, then you've surely found a means of "playing" on a daily basis.

However, for most Americans this is not the case. Not only do more than two-thirds of us work at jobs we dislike, we're also working harder than we used to. According to the Washington-based Economic Policy Institute, the average American works 158 hours more (including the increase in commuting time and the decrease in paid days off) every year than we did twenty years ago. That's the equivalent of an extra month of work. As our amount of leisure time has dwindled, we have become over-worked and overstressed by the joint demands of work and family life. We had an average of 16.1 days off a year in 1989, down from 19.8 days in 1981. In most European countries, workers get *paid vacations of at least five weeks.* Not surprisingly, the increased costs of health care and housing, along with the decline in real wages since 1973, are the major factors behind our need to put in more hours.

Whether or not you consider yourself overworked or have been able to experience work as play, I suggest that you find at least one activity other than work that you thoroughly enjoy. America is a recreational paradise. Even so, there are still many adults who have never given themselves the opportunity to play.

I recommend sports, games, dance, and other activities requiring some body movement, or active creative pursuits such as playing a musical instrument, acting, singing, painting, crafts, or gardening. Although I realize that many people derive great pleasure from playing cards or chess and other board games and from collecting stamps or coins, all these are mental exercises. In our society, we already spend most of our time exercising our minds. To create a healthier balance, we should be looking for activities that utilize our bodies, allow us to better express our feelings and creativity, and perhaps even bring us to a greater level of spiritual attunement. Ideally the activity should be something so consuming and absorbing that it requires total attention. In that way it provides a pleasurable escape from our normal tension and stress and habitual thoughts.

If you played little as a child, or never developed a hobby or strong interest in any particular recreational activity, choose something that instinctively appeals to you. Then find a good teacher or a class and learn the basics. Be prepared to make mistakes and look silly. That's part of the risk of doing something new. After that first step (always the most difficult one), it will be a matter of making a commitment and practicing. The better you become, the more you'll enjoy and appreciate the benefits of the activity. If you are not interested in learning something new, I suggest a simple activity such as walking or hiking. What's important is to choose something and do it on a regular basis, for at least one hour three times a week.

The importance of play cannot be overemphasized. We live in a culture where work has become the greatest addiction; where for many, achievement, accomplishment, and net financial worth determine self-worth. In such an environment, attaining a sense of wholeness and balance requires that we regularly, and for at least a short time, let go of that responsible, mature, working adult and get back in touch with our playful "inner child."

EMOTIONAL CAUSES OF DIS-EASE

Every disease has multiple causes. There is often a genetic predisposition to developing a chronic ailment that is inherited from parents and grandparents. The risk of contracting cancer or heart disease is increased significantly if one or both parents has it. My father and one of my daughters has chronic sinusitis. Allergies also commonly run in families.

As you've learned in chapters 7 and 8, environmental and dietary factors also play important roles in the disease process.

But before an acute illness can continue to progress into a chronic condition, there must be an accompanying diminished function of the immune system. After being sick for a short time, normal immune function restores the body to its original state of good health.

In most cases, the primary cause of chronically depressed immunity is emotional stress. "Stress" is a broad and ubiquitous term in our "stressed out" society—stress management, stress reduction, stress-ful. Most of us recognize that stress doesn't feel good if there's too much of it, but what actually causes it? The answer to that question is different for each of us. But how many of us are actually able to identify the specific emotion most responsible for our feelings of stress? Are you depressed, angry, ashamed, guilty, afraid, or sad?

Holistic physicians and researchers in behavioral medicine and psychoneuroimmunology are just beginning to connect consistent emotional and behavioral patterns with predictable dis-ease responses. With chronic respiratory disease, I have mentioned the critical role of repressed anger in causing chronic sinusitis. Many of my sinus patients are high achievers with a strong need for control. Anger is often a result of their perceived loss of control. I also now believe that a deep sadness exists in most of these patients. The many tears that have not been shed can result in congestion of the tear glands that surround the eyes and that are in close proximity to the sinuses as well. Perhaps this swelling and congestion is also a contributor to congested sinuses.

Besides the skin tests and a scientific investigation of their environment to determine the cause of hay fever, people with allergies would do well to ask themselves who or what situation or circumstance they are "allergic" to. For several years I have been increasingly aware of the intimate connection between sneezing spells and disturbing thoughts or images. One patient in particular, who was having marital problems, would start to sneeze whenever I mentioned her husband. Yes, of course the pollen count or cat dander are certainly contributors. But even with those factors being present, symptoms can be minimal or nonexistent until a disturbing thought or situation occurs. Then the feeling of stress arises, and the allergy attack begins. The next time you experience a sudden onset of allergy symptoms, I would suggest looking back to your thoughts and feelings that were present just prior to the allergic reaction. Your sneezing, itching, congestion, and wheezing can become an emotional "barometer" that helps you to identify the deeper and hidden causes of allergic rhinitis and asthma.

For many children with asthma there is excessive enmeshment, a smothering love, between parent and child. This overpowering relationship can create a feeling of being stifled and a degree of dependence that nearly equates with the child's inability to breathe for himself. Asthma is also often associated with suppressed crying. The underlying emotional factors with bronchitis are very similar to those with sinusitis.

I recognize that I have made a generalization regarding the emotional causes of respiratory diseases, and that they do not apply to everyone with these conditions. But before promptly dismissing them as not pertaining to you, please give it some thought and try to identify what it is you are feeling.

Another method you might use to help identify the emotional causes of your illness is to consider the possible benefits or secondary gain resulting from being sick. This is most easily seen with colds, which usually occur during a period when you've often been working too hard or doing too much. The cold might necessitate staying home in bed, missing a day of work, and receiving a lot more nurturing—all of which were sorely needed. Since you did not respond preventively, in order to meet those unconscious needs your body created an illness. Whether it's more attention, a need to be cared for, job dissatisfaction, or school phobia, I believe there are always secondary gains associated with every chronic disease. If these not so subtle benefits can be understood, they can help you to recognize the emotional causes of your physical problem. Once you have become aware of these emotions, you can then begin the process of accepting (knowing that it's okay to feel whatever you're feeling) and expressing all of your feelings and addressing the unmet needs your feelings bring up. This process will not only lead you to emotional health, it will also take you a giant step closer to being completely free of your so called "incurable" dis-ease.

EMOTIONAL HEALTH RECOMMENDATIONS: A SUMMARY

- Love and fear: These are the two basic human emotions. All other feelings are aspects of these. The more of one you feel, the less you'll feel of the other.
- Mental/emotional overlap: Unhealthy, negative emotions, such as depression and anxiety, are frequently caused by illogical, distorted, and unrealistic thoughts.
- Psychotherapy: Choose a psychotherapist carefully from among a group of mental health professionals that include psychiatrists, psychologists, holistic physicians, social workers, pastoral counselors, and those with degrees in counseling. Be clear on your objectives before beginning.
- Meditation: This involves conscious breathing, with benefits in every realm of holistic health. Start with five minutes twice a day and gradually increase to twenty minutes.
- Breath therapy: Any one of a number of methods based on conscious breathing may be used. They help uncover deeply held emotions. The method should be learned from a breath therapist.
- Dream interpretation: The very process of remembering a dream promotes emotional stability. Record dreams in writing or with a tape recorder as soon as you awaken.
- Journaling: Keeping a daily written record of your thoughts and feelings will help you to become your own therapist and best friend.
- Emotional release: Practice at least one anger release technique daily. Most are physical methods that include screaming, punching, hitting, and stamping. Crying can improve your mood, release tension, and remove toxins from the body.
- Play: Select a sport, game, activity, or creative pursuit requir-

ing body movement. Try to practice it for one hour three times a week. Allow yourself to become more childlike.

- Emotional causes: Pay more attention to your feelings at the beginning of and, especially, *just before* the start of a cold, sinus infection, allergy or asthma attack. Try to understand what benefits you might derive from being sick.
- Remember, *if you can't feel it, you can't heal it.*

Chapter 12

SPIRITUAL HEALTH

I want to make it clear that this discussion of spiritual health is not a discourse on religion, although it is based on truths common to all religions. To me, spiritual health means a heightened awareness of a power greater than oneself. This power can be referred to as God, the Creator, the Source, Infinite Intelligence, Jesus, Adonai, Yahweh, Allah, or your inner healer, voice, teacher, guide, child, or higher self. Whatever term feels most comfortable to you is the right one. A program of spiritual fitness will balance the metaphysical with the material, giving you more access to this higher power. The result will be a profound reduction in your feelings of fear and an increased capacity to love both yourself and others unconditionally. Additional benefits might include reversing heart disease (spiritual health is an integral part of Dr. Dean Ornish's treatment program) and eliminating substance abuse (spirituality is the basis of the Twelve-Step programs used for alcohol, drug, and other addictions). A spiritual fitness program is also great for healing sick sinuses!

Each of the world's great religions prescribes a method for gaining greater awareness of God. Each religion believes that it is the one correct path to spiritual enlightenment. All of these faiths express their essence in a single moral principle:

Buddhism: *Hurt not others in ways that you yourself would find hurtful.*

UDANAVARGA 5:18

Christianity: *All things whatsoever you would that men should do to you, do ye even so to them.*

MATTHEW 7:12

Confucianism: *Do not unto others what you would not have them do unto you.*

ANALECTS 15:23

Hinduism: *Do naught unto others which would cause you pain if done to you.*

MAHABHARATA 5:1517

Islam: *No one of you is a believer until he desires for his brother that which he desires for himself.*

SUNAN

Judaism: *Thou shalt love thy neighbor as thyself.*

LEVITICUS 19:18

Judaism: *What is hateful to you, do not to your fellow man.*

TALMUD, CHABBAT 31A

An equally important objective of most of these religions is that the believer love God or come to know God. The essence of the Judeo-Christian doctrine is expressed in the words that Jewish people are instructed to repeat thrice daily, "You shall love the Lord your God, with all your heart, with all your soul, and with all your might."

What hasn't been quite so clear to most of us is *how* one loves God. Some have found their answer by living in harmony with nature. James Lovelock, Ph.D., in his book *The Ages of Gaia: A Biography of Our Living Earth,* describes our planet and everything on it as a single living organism. He believes that the dynamic forces that have shaped the globe for the past 4.5 billion years are still modifying the environment to allow the survival of all life forms and that this process is guided by an intrinsic homeostatic mechanism. People who live close to the earth recognize this guiding intelligence as God. Its essence is found not only in the earth, but in themselves and every other living organism on the planet. This life force is referred to as chai (pronounced "hi") in Hebrew, chi in Chinese, and ki in Japanese. Interestingly, our culture does not have a comparable word. This life force is the core spiritual component of every human being and our common bond with our Creator, the earth, our fellow human beings, and all other life forms.

For many people in today's urban technological society, however, God is now found in science. These people have lost any sense of proximity or harmony with the earth, along with the awareness that technology is contributing to its destruction. They expect science to provide them with food and water, stimulate their minds, entertain them, allow them to exercise conveniently, solve most urban problems, fix the environmental crisis it has created, and also heal our diseased bodies. However, science is restricted to the material world, one that can only be experienced through our five physical senses: sight, hearing, touch, taste, and smell. Science is the world of effect. Beyond it, in the realm of the metaphysical, lies cause. *Metaphysics,* defined in Webster's *New World Dictionary* as "the branch of philosophy that deals with first principles and seeks to explain the nature of being or reality and the origin and structure of the world," refers to ideas and concepts beyond the scope of our five senses.

Science believes that the universe is ordered and that it obeys the law of cause and effect; e.g., for every action there is an equal and opposite reaction. However, scientific method on its own is incapable of generating new ideas. In *Where Is Science Going?,* physicist Max Planck wrote, "When the pioneer in science sends forth the groping fingers of his thoughts, he must have a vivid, intuitive imagination, for new ideas are not generated by deduction, but by an artistically creative imagination." In the field of health, psychoneuroimmunology, a product of this type of creative thinking, is building a solid scientific bridge between the world of the physical and the world of the metaphysical. I am hoping that this book will enable you to walk across that bridge with me.

Our modern lifestyle has created a distance between humanity and the earth's natural rhythms. Yet our spiritual essence, the divine spark or life force energy within each of us, is transcendent and connects us to all of creation. This concept has been repeated throughout history by almost every prophet and spiritual teacher of every religion. Jesus put it most succinctly: "The kingdom of God is within." I believe that in contemporary society *the simplest and most effective way to learn to love God is to learn to love yourself.*

The "self" I am referring to is not exactly the one you have come to know. Many of us spend our lives confusing our traits, habits, and actions with ourselves. "This is who I am," we say. Psychology refers to this sense of self as the ego, our conscious personality. We spend almost all of our waking time in the ego, and it constitutes much of the mental and emotional aspects of the self. However, there is still far more to a human being than these components. W. Brugh Joy, M.D., a pioneer in holistic medicine and the author of *Joy's Way* and *Avalanche—Heretical Reflections on the Dark and the Light,* offers the analogy of the human ego as a subatomic particle on the tip of a hair on the tail of a dog, wagging the dog. An entire person, including the spiritual component, encompasses a great deal more than the human intellect can comprehend. There are, however, many ways to explore these vast realms of your unconscious and discover a much deeper sense of love and appreciation for the unique individual that you really are. This process can result in a greater degree of unconditional love for yourself and others, and in that feeling lies an experience of God or a power greater than yourself. What follows are several methods to assist you on this enlivening journey. To help clarify my own goal of spiritual health, I often repeat to myself this saying by the late Teilhard de Chardin, a former priest: "Joy is the most infallible sign of the presence of God!"

MEANING, PURPOSE, AND INTUITION

If you have ever asked yourself the question, "Who am I?," "Where am I going?," or "What am I here to do?," you have already begun your spiritual journey. These questions often arise spontaneously as a result of a heightened sense of mortality, as with advancing age or with a chronic or terminal disease. But many who seek to better understand the meaning of their lives are neither old nor sick. They might have attained their life's goals, or realized the American Dream, a vision that embraces society's values of financial success, power, and public recognition. Having achieved "all anyone could ever want," they often find it a hollow success. They feel an emptiness that begs the questions: "Is that all there is to life?"; "Now what?"; "Isn't there anything more?" Until now, their life's meaning had been defined by society, a definition that was imposed externally rather than one that came from within.

For me, the answers began to unfold when I encountered the work of Elisabeth Kübler-Ross, M.D. This remarkable psychiatrist has been investigating the phenomena of death and dying for most of her career, perhaps longer than any other member of the medical community. Kübler-Ross has concluded from her many years of research that "death does not exist"! She believes that what we call death is merely the shedding of a physical shell housing an immortal spirit, that our time spent in these bodies on earth is but a very brief part of the total span of our existence, and that *to live well while we are here means to learn to love.*

Initially I was stunned by her words. This was medical science's leading authority on the one subject that most unnerves physicians—who are trained to equate death with failure—and she was making what sounded like some very unscientific remarks. I was unable to dismiss them, however, and in the eleven years since learning of her conclusions, I have confirmed for myself their validity. Believing in the existence of spirit and recognizing love as a means of gaining access to its healing potential have helped me to transform not only my medical practice but my life as well. This perspective has provided me with a new direction, goals, and values; it has reduced dramatically my fear of death and enriched my life beyond measure.

Each of us responds differently. An answer that might inspire a greater sense of meaning and direction for one might do nothing for another. What is most important is that you begin asking the questions. If you have taken that first step, as long as you are patient you'll find what you're looking for. The answers might not come like bolts of lightning, but perhaps like a light controlled by a dimmer switch, gradually illuminating a dark or unexplored aspect of your mind. Your guide along this new path will be your intuition. I have heard this inner voice described as "God talking to you." Your progress on this journey of change will be determined by the degree to which you trust your intuition.

The quiet, subtle messages from your intuition have a tough time competing for your attention. Most of the inner messages you hear come from your ego and are loud, often negative, and based on fear. However, if you learn to listen, you will begin to hear a "still, small voice" from the depths of your awareness. If you are interested in developing your sense of intuition, you will have to slow down, eliminate distractions, and do a lot less talking. Meditation, conscious breathing, and slow, relaxing (not brisk, exercise-oriented) walks are all helpful methods of learning to listen to this inner voice.

Learning to follow your intuition is both a life-changing adventure and an enlivening exercise that strengthens your life energy. Just as with any other type of exercise, practice is required. The more you can follow that "hunch" or "gut instinct" or "deep inner voice" and get results that feel good to you, the more you will trust it. This is the foundation upon which faith is built—faith in oneself, God, and the universe. It can become the basis for the belief that the world is really a safe and loving place, where it is okay to trust. If you can learn to trust your intuition, this trust can then extend to the way you interact with the world and can dramatically reduce the amount of stress in your life. This doesn't mean that you will ignore known risks to your health, safety, and security, but it will offer a means of minimizing fear.

There will be instances in which you believe you have been following your intuition and yet the results are painful. You quit your old job only to find less satisfaction with the new one, you move to a new home that turns out to create a lot more headaches than the one you left, or you divorce a spouse and marry someone else with whom you have similar conflicts. These are not necessarily mistakes. They can be seen as lessons. When we were students and failed to learn a subject, we were given a chance to repeat the course. Life can present lessons to us in much the same way, and often painfully.

If you are questioning the meaning of your life, it can be helpful to look back at some of your most painful experiences. Look at the role you played in each one and how you might have contributed to the situation. Ask yourself if there were recognizable patterns of behavior. For example, I have been treating a patient for chronic back pain, which at times has incapacitated her. Before the first attack, her life was a whirlwind of activity— mother, housewife, PTA, sales job, and aerobics instructor. The back pain made it nearly impossible for her to continue with any of her former responsibilities. As soon as it had subsided, however, she resumed her hectic pace, and within a year the problem had returned. This time it was worse, and it put her out of commission for nearly three months. During this period of inactivity, while lying on her back, she began to understand her overwhelming desire to achieve and her strong need to give to others. Without her achievements or the ability to give, she felt worthless. Like so many Americans, she did not feel entitled to love unless she was accomplishing at a high level or taking care of others. She gave very little to herself. Rather than taking the time to learn and appreciate what it means to be a human being, she had become a human "doing," and quite a good one at that.

Her back has been much better for nearly two years, and she has developed a lifestyle that is much more gentle, nurturing, and healthy. She gives more to herself, works only part-time, and, as a result, is able to spend more time with her family. From this experience she has developed a much greater degree of trust in her intuition, as it directs her on a path of caring for herself with more compassion. Facing an exceptionally painful situation with forgiveness and acceptance rather than anger and fear will bring greater meaning to your life and give you an opportunity to grow spiritually. *Man's Search for Meaning* by Viktor Frankl, M.D., a survivor of a Nazi concentration camp, is an inspirational book on this subject.

Others find greater meaning by conducting their lives as if they have very little time left to live. In his book on spiritual health, *The Road Less Traveled,* M. Scott Peck, M.D., describes the benefits of living with "death on your left shoulder." This approach quickly and dramatically puts life into a different perspective. It forces you to reexamine your values and decide what is really important.

Whatever route you take, as you look for meaning in life you will usually discover greater purpose. Every individual has at least one unique talent or God-given gift. Often it is in the expression of this gift that one finds purpose. To me, one's purpose is to share his or her gift and, as a result, leave the world a better place. I know of no more effective way to realize your purpose than working on a personalized program of holistic health. Several of my student/patients have realized that their gift is for healing, a discovery that has caused them to redirect their professional careers. Some of life's greatest joys come from practicing your gifts and doing what you love to do. Getting paid for doing it can be an added bonus.

PRAYER

Prayer is both a spiritual exercise and the standard Western form of meditation. A Gallup poll in 1988 found that 88 percent of

Americans pray. Most of those who do pray have a greater sense of well-being than those who don't. A majority said that they experience a sense of peace when they pray, have received answers to their prayers, and have felt divinely inspired or "led by God" to perform some specific action. Those who said they felt an experience of the divine during prayer are the people who have the highest rating in general well-being or satisfaction with their lives. More than 70 percent of Americans believe prayer can lead to physical, emotional, or spiritual healing.

In a study conducted by Randolph Byrd, M.D., at the San Francisco General Medical Center, Christians were asked to pray for half of a group of 393 hospitalized heart disease patients; no one was assigned to pray for the other half. The patients were unaware of which group they were in. The results showed that a majority of those who were prayed for needed less medical intervention during their hospital stay than those in the control group.

Herbert Benson, M.D., a Harvard cardiologist, has been conducting research that has conclusively demonstrated that prayer benefits health. He began his research in 1968, using subjects who practiced transcendental meditation. They meditated with a mantra, a single word with no meaning to its user, such as *om.* Dr. Benson found that repetition of the mantra replaced the arousing thoughts that otherwise kept them tense during most waking hours. This resulted in a lower metabolic rate, slower heart rate, lower blood pressure, and slower breathing.

Dr. Benson then studied Christians and Jews who prayed rather than meditated. He asked Roman Catholic subjects to repeat "Hail Mary, full of grace" or "Lord Jesus Christ, have mercy upon me." Jews used "Shalom," the peace greeting, or "Echad," meaning "one." Protestants used the first line of the Lord's Prayer, "Our Father, who art in heaven," or the opening of Psalm 23, "The Lord is my shepherd." The phrases all had the same physiological effect as the meditation. Dr. Benson has found that all major religious traditions use simple repetitive prayers. Such repetitions, his research suggests, create what he calls the relaxation response (RR). This response is the opposite of the stress reaction widely known as the flight-or-fight response: in human beings, the physical reaction to perceived danger.

As he continued his studies, Dr. Benson found that faith affects the physiological benefits of RR and that prayer initiates the response. He also found a connection between RR and exercise: when runners meditated or prayed as they ran, their bodies were more efficient. They were able to achieve even greater efficiency by matching the cadence of their short prayers to the rhythm of their stride.

Since 1988, Dr. Benson and psychologist Jared Kass have been conducting a series of programs at the Mind/Body Medical Institute at Boston's New England Deaconess Hospital. They have invited priests, ministers, and rabbis to investigate the spiritual and health implications of prayer. *They found that people who feel themselves in touch with God are less likely to get sick—and better able to cope when they do.* Drs. Benson and Kass developed a psychological scale for measuring spirituality both before and after prayer. Those high in spirituality, which Benson defines as the feeling that "there is more than just you" and as not necessarily religious, scored high in psychological health. They also have fewer stress-related symptoms. Next, he found that people high in spirituality gain the most from meditation training; they show the greatest rise on a life-purpose index as well as the sharpest drop in pain. The nearly three-quarters of the American population who already believe that prayer can be therapeutic now have additional confirmation: science has shown that as prayer strengthens the spirit, it can also heal the body.

For those of you who already pray, I recommend that you continue. For those who would like to begin, I suggest you start with any prayer with which you might be comfortable or can remember from your religious training. The Lord's Prayer is familiar to most Christians, and the majority of Jews know the Shema and Viahavta. Try to establish a regular routine and repeat the prayer morning and night. You might have a favorite psalm or a passage from the Bible or a prayer book that is especially meaningful. Add it to your daily regimen. I have found three psalms in particular to be especially healing: 121, which I repeat every morning; 91, which I say in late afternoons or after work; and 23, which I say before bed.

In addition to the prayers and psalms associated with religion and the Bible, you might be interested in more personal prayer. To do this, talk to God as if you are speaking to your best friend. Be extremely honest; for example, "I'm having a problem and I really need some help." It is fine to want material things or health for yourself or loved ones, but first ask yourself what feeling would result from having the things for which you ask. I suggest praying for that feeling rather than the specific things.

In an experiment performed by the Spindrift organization in Lansdale, Pennsylvania, the effectiveness of directed and nondirected prayer was tested. Those practicing directed prayer had a specific goal, image, or outcome in mind, while nondirected prayer is an open-ended approach in which no specific outcome is held in the mind. The practitioner of nondirected prayer does not attempt "to tell the universe what to do." The results proved conclusively that chances are much greater for attaining the desired outcome when one prays only for "what's best"—"Thy will be done."

Larry Dossey, M.D., former co-chairman of the Panel on Mind/Body Interventions, Office of Alternative Medicine at the National Institutes of Health, has written several excellent books related to the subject of prayer and healing. They are *Healing Words; Meaning and Medicine;* and *Recovering the Soul.*

GRATITUDE

Most religious traditions prescribe specific prayers or grace before meals as a means of thanking God for the food and for our physical sustenance. As with other spiritual practices, there is something to be gained from these rituals, or they wouldn't have survived for thousands of years. The more you can appreciate the spirit of the practice rather than merely following its form, the greater its value will be. Science is just beginning to appreciate the multifaceted benefits of spirituality.

Feelings of gratitude can elicit similar life-enhancing benefits. One of the most spiritual rabbis I have ever met suggests this ritual: As soon as you wake up each morning, even before getting out of bed, close your eyes and picture yourself in a scene that made you happy to be alive and for which you are still grateful to have experienced. You never would have had that experience if you weren't living, and you know that something equally wonderful can happen again. What a great way to instill an attitude of anticipation and appreciation for being alive and to begin the new day.

Most of us tend to take life for granted. Suppose you choose instead to see your life as a gift, to be thankful for all that it has provided you—both the pleasure and the pain. Adversity can give you the opportunity for tremendous growth. You might not be too happy about it at the time, but in retrospect you can be grateful for the lessons you've learned.

Gratitude can produce powerful feelings of joy and self-acceptance. It is an attitude that anyone can choose to have, just as you can choose to be positive or negative, be forgiving or unforgiving, see the cup as half full or half empty. It has been my experience that when people choose to look at the up side of life, more positive things start to happen. It seems that we attract whatever feeling we radiate. When you focus on gratitude, wonderful things happen. When you focus on what you do have, not on what you don't have, you feel a sense of abundance, which enables you to let go of negative thoughts and attitudes.

This isn't easy to do. If you are feeling a great deal of fear and anger, it is especially difficult to superimpose gratitude, but if you can release some of those feelings through forgiveness and acceptance and put your heart into practicing gratitude, I know it will work for you.

As long as you are alive blessings will come your way. I rarely go through a day without thanking God for something, and every time I do there is an accompanying feeling of joy.

SPIRITUAL PRACTICES

Most major religions have their own variations on the following practices, but none of them needs to be performed in accordance with any particular ritual in order to be enjoyed. Doing them in whatever way is comfortable for you, or even creating your own ritual, will feel good. These basic practices involve fasting, the Sabbath, and the four fundamental elements of our world: earth, air, fire, and water.

Earth

Nature can give us a feeling of proximity to God and a healing energy that can't be found in most congested urban environments. I recommend spending as much time as possible outdoors in close contact with the earth, or at least in natural settings— parks, woods, beaches, or mountains. A daily walk is great, or playing a sport, riding your bike, swimming—especially in the ocean, a lake, or a river—gardening, or just finding a quiet or scenic spot to appreciate the surrounding beauty.

In 1981 Roger Ulrich, Ph.D., a professor of urban and regional planning at Texas A&M, performed a study with the help of Swedish scientists. He showed eighteen students slides of trees, plants, water, and cities. The students reported that the nature scenes, especially those of water, made them feel more elated and relaxed; in contrast, the urban scenes tended to elicit sadness and fear. Electroencephalograph (EEG) readings of the students' brain-wave activity showed significantly stronger alpha waves when viewing the nature scenes—scientific evidence of feelings of relaxed wakefulness.

In 1984 Dr. Ulrich found that exposure to nature speeds recovery from the stress of surgery. When he examined the hospital records of forty-six men and women who had undergone gallbladder operations, those with a window view of a small grove of trees were hospitalized about a day less than patients with a view of a brick wall. They also required less pain medication and were less upset.

Air

Find a place to meditate where the air is reasonably healthy. See the Meditation and Breathing Therapy section in Chapter 11 for specifics on meditation.

Fire

Throughout the Bible, the dominant symbol for the divine essence in man is fire or light. Anyone who enjoys camping can attest to the pleasure of an open fire. A fireplace at home offers the same satisfaction, but because wood burning contributes to air pollution and sinus problems, I recommend a gas fireplace. The simplest and healthiest choice is to enjoy candlelight whenever possible.

Water

I have already emphasized the importance of drinking plenty of water. Now I am suggesting that you immerse yourself in it. There is nothing quite so relaxing as bathing in warm water. I suggest doing it at least once a day, morning or night. Hot tubs and spas are two of technology's greatest inventions, but if you don't have either, a bathtub will suffice. If you have ever soaked in a natural outdoor hot spring, congratulations—you have experienced what I consider one of life's ultimate pleasures. Mineral hot springs can be therapeutic for a variety of ailments. In some that are unimproved (without a cement foundation), you can at times feel so close to nature that it is almost as if you are floating in the womb of Mother Earth.

Fasting

The ancient ritual of purification by abstaining from food can have a cleansing effect upon the body. According to the Bible, Moses and Jesus were both able to sustain fasts for forty days. Unless you have attained their level of spiritual mastery, please don't attempt a fast of that duration. I recommend one day, during which you abstain from both food and water. Doing this can definitely elicit a heightened spiritual feeling, as your focus shifts away from physical concerns. Select a day when work and family responsibilities are limited and you won't be too active. Plan for some quiet time alone, and during the final two hours of the fast drink six to eight glasses of water. This helps to cleanse your body of toxins. See how it feels after you have fasted once or twice, and if you think it has been beneficial, try fasting on a regular basis, perhaps monthly. You will be surprised at how much easier it is with each subsequent fast.

Sabbath

"Remember the Sabbath day to keep it holy." Although more than 3,000 years old, the Ten Commandments remain a worthy set of ethics. To the Jewish people, the Sabbath is still the holiest day on the calendar, even though it occurs every week. It is meant to be a day completely devoted to love—of God, self, family, and friends. I am not suggesting that you observe any particular day of the week or even a full day if you can't afford the time. For your spiritual health, however, I recommend setting aside the same time each week to indulge yourself in this celebration of life. Try to abstain from anything even remotely resembling work.

Eye Contact

Looking at yourself, especially your eyes, in a mirror for five minutes every day can be a very powerful exercise. It works best to look into your left eye, which is connected to the more "receptive" right side of your brain. Doing this practice on a daily basis can help you learn to love what you see. Louise Hay recommends that while doing this mirror work you say, "I love me." This spiritual exercise will also make it easier to make eye contact with others, as well as being able to tell them, "I love you."

Touch

There are several topics that don't fit easily into one single component of holistic health but that offer several healing benefits simultaneously. Touch is one of them. I have included it here because it is not only one of our most effective healers, it might well be the most powerful and direct means of conveying love.

According to Saul Schanberg, M.D., Ph.D., a professor of pharmacology and biological psychiatry at Duke University, "Humans need to touch and be touched, just as we need food and water." His research and that of other experts on touch were cited in *Hands-on Healing,* edited by John Feltman.

- In a study involving forty premature infants, half of them were gently stroked for forty-five minutes a day; the other twenty were not. Although all were fed the same amount of calories, after ten days, the touched babies weighed in 47 percent heavier than the unstimulated group. The stroked babies were also more active, more alert, and more responsive to social stimulation.
- When a person's wrist is gently held by someone else, the heartbeat slows and blood pressure declines.
- Children and adolescents hospitalized for psychiatric problems show remarkable reductions in anxiety levels and positive changes in attitude when they receive a brief daily back rub.
- The arteries of rabbits fed a high-cholesterol diet and petted regularly had 60 percent less blockage than did the arteries of unpetted but similarly fed rabbits.
- Rats that were handled for fifteen minutes a day during the first three weeks of their lives showed dramatically less

cell deterioration and memory loss as they grew old, compared with nonhandled rats.

Yet in spite of the many healthy reasons to touch and be touched by other human beings, Americans indulge very little in this simple pleasure. One study in the 1960s noted the number of touches exchanged by pairs of people sitting in coffee shops around the world. In San Juan, Puerto Rico, people touched 180 times an hour; in Paris, France, 110 times an hour; in Gainesville, Florida, 2 times an hour; and in London, England, the pairs never touched. The implications and possible causes of this phenomenon would entail a lengthy discussion, although I am sure the puritanical legacy of associating touch with sex has had a profound effect on American attitudes. William E. Whitehead, Ph.D., an associate professor of medical psychology at the Johns Hopkins University School of Medicine, believes that a significant part of the blame lies with the father of modern-day psychology, Sigmund Freud. "Freud encouraged austerity in dealing with children. And parents bought into that behavior," says Dr. Whitehead. People who aren't cuddled a lot as kids, he adds, tend to develop into nontouching adults. The cycle then repeats itself, generation after generation.

As an osteopathic physician, I learned very early in my medical training about the therapeutic value of the "laying on of hands." Although almost all of our courses and textbooks were the same as those used to train allopathic medical doctors (M.D.s), we were also taught a holistic approach to health care that included osteopathic manipulative therapy. Soft-tissue stretching (somewhat similar to massage) and adjustments or corrections in the position of the spine and other body parts (similar to chiropractic adjustments) are part of this therapy. It has taken me a while to realize that patients responded well to this treatment not only because of the prescribed techniques, but also because of the healing potential of the touch itself. I have learned since of other therapies in which touch is a primary healing ingredient. They are acupressure, the Alexander technique, applied kinesiology, Aston-patterning, the Berry method, chiropractic, craniosacral therapy, Esalen massage, the Feldenkrais method, Hellerwork, hydrotherapy, myotherapy, oriental massage, physiatry, physical therapy, polarity therapy, reflexology, Reichian therapy, Rolfing, sports massage, Swedish massage, therapeutic touch, and the Trager approach. I will not discuss the relative merits of these methods other than to say that all of them deserve to be recognized as legitimate disciplines in the full spectrum of the healing arts.

I have always viewed the practice of medicine as the business of caring. As our health care system continues to change radically, the most insidious shift has been the erosion of the doctor-patient relationship. As it becomes more impersonal, there is less mutual trust. Within the conventional medical community there is a greater fear of closeness, which leads to limiting the touching of patients to that which is strictly necessary in the course of a diagnostic evaluation. Sick people need the comfort of human touch more than healthy people—a reassuring pat on the shoulder, hand-holding, or even a hug. If caregivers are to do their best job, this powerful method of healing must be learned. Touch has to become a larger component of every physician's therapeutic black bag.

If you are interested in experiencing a hands-on healing technique, I suggest trying a practitioner of one of the many therapies previously mentioned. See how it feels and give it a fair trial. If it works for you, that's great. If it doesn't, try something else. In my experience three of these, acupressure, cranial osteopathy, and reflexology, have been effective in treating chronic sinusitis. They are described in Chapter 14.

Touch is a gift you can give to yourself every day. It requires allowing yourself to receive and to feel deserving. If you are meditating, praying, or lying in the bathtub, try touching your chest over your heart in as gentle and compassionate a way as you know how. A loving touch is healing, no matter who gives it.

Animals are perfectly fine sources of tactile comfort, says Alan M. Beck, Sc.D., director of the Center for the Interaction of Animals and Society at the University of Pennsylvania. Numerous studies, he adds, "definitely show that petting an animal can lower one's blood pressure.'' Other doctors suggest that there are health benefits to be had even from cuddling inanimate objects—teddy bears, for instance. If you have neither a pet nor a favorite stuffed animal, my prescription for maintaining your spiritual health is to get several hugs daily!

There is no question that we have become too distant from one another. There is clearly a movement in this country to compensate for that deficiency and restore our sense of wholeness and balance. The trend toward more touching is a return to the norms and values of preindustrialized society. Primitive cultures are all very touch oriented. I have lived with one such native group in which touch is their primary method of healing. These people believe that their healers have a gift bestowed by God, and that the healing energy that flows through the healer to the patient is God's love. Whatever its source, the healers' touch works extremely well for a variety of ailments. By our standards these people might be considered primitive or underdeveloped, but they are clearly much healthier than most Americans in body, mind, and spirit.

SPIRITUAL HEALTH RECOMMENDATIONS: A SUMMARY

- Spirituality is *awareness of a power greater than yourself,* most commonly referred to as God. This divine power is the essence of all life on earth and is the spark or life force energy within every human being.
- *Knowing or loving God and loving your neighbor as yourself* are the primary moral principles of most religions. As spiritual health objectives in contemporary American society, they can best be reached through first learning to love yourself. As you do, you will experience less fear in your life and a deeper sense of unconditional love for yourself and others. In that feeling lies a greater awareness of God.
- *Meaning, purpose, and intuition:* Begin by asking yourself what your life is about, where you're heading, and what you enjoy

doing. This will help clarify your sense of purpose as well as provide the opportunity to give your gifts to others. Your intuition, or inner voice, is your best guide in the process. Take time to listen and be willing to risk in learning to trust it.

- *Prayer:* Daily prayers, those prescribed from your religious training or personalized "talking to God" prayers, are helpful. I also recommend Psalm 121 in the morning, Psalm 91 after work, and Psalm 23 before bed.

- *Gratitude:* Begin your day by visualizing a scene that makes you feel happy to be alive. Don't take life for granted; there are numerous blessings for which to be grateful. Focus on what you have, not on what you lack.

- *Spiritual practices:* Use the four basic elements of our world by engaging in outdoor activities that enhance closeness to the earth, meditating or using conscious breathing somewhere with clean air, using candles more often, and soaking daily in a warm bath, hot tub, or natural hot spring. Fasting for one day periodically and observing a regular weekly Sabbath (a day to focus on love, for yourself and others) are both effective practices.

- *Touch:* This is a basic human need that for most of us is filled far too seldom. There are many therapeutic disciplines in which touch is the primary attribute. If you are treating a chronic condition that has not responded to your present regimen, consider choosing one of these approaches. Remember, too, that hugs heal!

Chapter 13

SOCIAL HEALTH

Social health comes from connections to other human beings. It requires the balance of autonomy with intimacy. I have found it to be the aspect of holistic health in which we Americans are most deficient, and it is clearly the most difficult for us to improve. The reasons for this social malaise are an ongoing topic for much discussion. I have no doubt that it was aggravated by the self-involvement of the seventies and the compelling profit motive, greed, and win-at-all-costs attitude of the eighties expressed by the bumper sticker "He who dies with the most toys wins."

The origin of this social disease might be debatable, but its impact on the family—the very foundation of social stability—is unmistakable. As a society we are feeling the pain of a pervasive sense of isolation: a 50 percent divorce rate, a general sentiment of feeling overworked, dual-career marriages, and a generation of children more adrift and alone than any that has preceded them. According to *Turning Points,* the 1989 report of the Carnegie Council on Adolescent Development, almost half of all adolescents are at significant risk of reaching adulthood unable to meet the requirements of the workplace, to make the commitments to family and friends, and to accept the responsibilities inherent in a democratic society. They are susceptible to "a vortex of new risks . . . almost unknown to their parents and grandparents."

Our young people reflect the world we have shaped for them. What seems dysfunctional in teenagers' behavior actually might be functional ways of dealing with the crazy environment they have inherited. What they reflect is our lack of connectedness with others. This sense of alienation can create both social and physical disease. Dean Ornish, M.D., a professor at the University of California School of Medicine at San Francisco, found that the common denominator among heart disease patients was their feeling of hostility and a sense of isolation. The importance of social relationships can also be seen in the high incidence of illness and death after the loss of a loved one or even a simple move to a new city, state, or country. In a study conducted by Kenneth Pelletier, Ph.D., a professor of both medicine and psychiatry at the University of California School of Medicine at San Francisco, on terminal cancer patients with long-term survival, one of the strongest indicators was their relatively high degree of social involvement. University of Michigan sociologist James House and his group of researchers concluded that social isolation is statistically just as dangerous as smoking, high blood pressure, high cholesterol, obesity, or lack of exercise.

I know of two studies that powerfully demonstrated to me the health benefits of social fitness and a strong sense of community. In the small town of Roseto, Pennsylvania, the citizens consumed what today would be considered a horrendously high-fat diet. They had been eating this way for several decades, into the mid-1960s, when Stewart Wolf, M.D., began studying the health histories of Roseto's inhabitants, most of whom are Italian immigrants. As a result of Dr. Wolf's findings, the town has become famous. Why? Because of its surprisingly low death rates. According to researchers, there is only one clear-cut explanation for this finding: the extraordinarily close-knit family and community ties amongst Roseto's residents.

The other study that got my attention was conducted by federal researchers, and the findings were published in November 1993 in the *Journal of the American Medical Association*. It showed that despite poverty, poor access to medical care, and a lack of health insurance, Hispanics are surprisingly less likely than whites to die of most of the major chronic diseases, including all forms of cancer, heart disease, and respiratory ailments. It found that with certain notable exceptions, including diabetes, liver disease, and homicide, the overall health outlook for Hispanics is significantly better than for whites. Some health experts, including former Surgeon General Coello Novello, a Latina who is the first woman to serve in that post, theorize that Hispanic culture—which frowns on drinking and smoking and promotes strong family values—helps keep that population healthy in spite of socioeconomic disadvantages. But most researchers cannot explain the findings and believe the reason for this health disparity between whites and Hispanics is still a mystery.

SUPPORT GROUPS

We humans are socially dependent animals, and the quality of our lives depends a great deal on our level of social integration. (A fascinating look at the human animal can be found in Desmond Morris's *The Naked Ape*.) Human babies have the longest infant dependency in the animal kingdom. A foal can run within hours of its birth; a kitten or puppy can leave its mother within two months. We humans are born helpless and stay dependent for years. If we don't bond and receive continual care, we die. Relatively little of our behavior is programmed at birth. Most of our learning, beliefs, attitudes, and worldview are shaped by an almost umbilical connection to our culture. The need to be a part of a social system does not diminish in adulthood; in fact, it becomes more elaborate. We look to society to provide food, shelter, goods, information, and health care. It is not surprising that we suffer when our link to others is broken. The recent scientific acknowledgment that support groups help people with chronic disease makes perfect sense. David Spiegel, M.D., conducted a study at Stanford University School of Medicine on women with metastatic breast cancer. All of the women received chemotherapy or radiation therapy. One half of them were in a support group that met weekly for one year. These women lived twice as long as those who were not in the support group. Whether a person has AIDS, multiple sclerosis, Parkinson's disease, or diabetes, there is a support group available in most urban communities. Even sinus sufferers have joined these ranks. I helped to create the SERI Sinus Sufferers Support System (S⁵) at the Solar Energy Research Institute (now called NREL—National Renewable Energy Laboratory) in Denver, the first sinus support group that has come to my attention.

There is a movement in America toward a greater sense of community. Small support groups for those sharing common values and goals are becoming much more commonplace. Men's groups, women's groups, and couples' groups, perhaps affiliated with a church or synagogue, are gathering all over the country, some for the purpose of enhancing spiritual growth, but all benefiting from the social connection. They meet regularly; some weekly, others twice a month, and some monthly. This is a positive and healthy indication of our nation's social recovery.

COMMITTED RELATIONSHIPS AND MARRIAGE

Marriage can be the most difficult, as well as the most rewarding, of all relationships. It can potentially become the most powerful spiritual practice in which we can engage. Most religions regard this bond between a man and a woman as a holy union. If humanity's fundamental moral principle is to "love thy neighbor as thyself," its practice begins not with the person living next door, but with the neighbor with whom we share our bed.

A healthy marriage incorporates all of the ingredients of holistic health, which is synonymous with learning to love. There is probably not a more effective vehicle for curing sinus and the other respiratory diseases than to work on your marriage or committed relationship. John Gottman, Ph.D., a professor of psychology at the University of Washington in Seattle, studied the interaction of couples on videotape. He found that a husband's contempt for his wife predicted, over time, the wife's susceptibility to illness. By counting the number of the husband's facial expressions of contempt for his wife, Gottman could accurately estimate the number of infectious diseases she would have over the next four years.

The key to success is commitment to each other and to your growth, both that of the individual and that of the relationship. Once that pact is made, you will begin to recognize that the relationship is an entity that is greater than the two of you. As Maggie Scarf wrote in her book *Intimate Partners,* "When space is provided within the system—space for changing, growing, being different over the course of time—marriage can be the most therapeutic of relationships, the fertile terrain which permits both partners to expand, flourish, and attain their full potentials." Change entails letting go of parts of yourself, and as you do, you will realize that in giving more to the relationship you are ultimately giving to yourself.

Marriage also promotes physical health. People who are single, divorced, or widowed are twice as likely to die prematurely as those who are married. This is particularly true of men. In October 1990 a study at the University of California, San Francisco, found that single men between the ages of 55 and 64 are twice as likely to die within ten years as married men their age. For women, it is not marriage so much as having social support that lends a longevity edge. Unmarried people also wind up in the hospital for mental disorders five to ten times as frequently. So before deciding to divorce, you might want to ask yourselves if you have done all you could do to save the relationship.

After more than twenty-seven years of marriage, my wife, Harriet, and I share with other couples what we have learned together. The recommendations that follow are distilled from the counseling the two of us have received; from the couples classes we teach; from Harriet's marriage and family therapy practice; from two insightful books, *Getting the Love You Want* by Harville Hendrix, Ph.D., and Maggie Scarf's *Intimate Partners;* and from our many years of working to make our own relationship a more conscious one. The following is a brief discussion of the methods and exercises we find helpful. If you are interested in making a deeper commitment to your relationship, I suggest you begin with marriage counseling. As with any new course of study, it doesn't hurt to find yourselves a good teacher.

Shared Vision

A vision is really a way of defining your mutual goals and focusing your energy on their attainment. Without a vision, your relationship can become directionless, and your problem-solving behavior will reflect a crisis orientation. You already might have completed your individual list of goals suggested in Chapter 10. Now each of you individually should write another in the form of affirmations in the present tense. These should be *positive,* short, descriptive, specific, and begin with "we." For example, "We trust each other," "We can safely express our anger toward each other," or "We are very affectionate and touch each other daily." The list might include statements relating to the way you feel about each other, where you live, how you play together, how you resolve conflicts, what your sex life is like, and anything else that applies to your situation. Before sharing your vision with your partner and creating a mutual vision list, prioritize in numerical order the items on your list. The next step is to begin combining lists by starting with the affirmations having the highest value and alternating between the two lists to form a composite vision. As you proceed you should try to combine similar sentences from both lists while capturing their essence. When you have completed this "mutual relationship vision," schedule a time every day to read it to each other, or record it on a cassette and listen to it together. Do this exercise daily for at least sixty days. This is just one of the sixteen exercises described in Dr. Hendrix's book. An accompanying workbook is available from his Institute for Relationship Therapy in New York City.

Listening Exercise

Most of us are very poor listeners. It amazes me at times how little we actually hear when we seem to be listening. Since communication is the foundation of any relationship, and listening is a critical aspect of effective communication, this exercise can go a long way toward creating greater intimacy and autonomy. It can also be good for your health. At the University of Maryland, James Lynch, Ph.D., found that people who do not listen well, who jump at the first chance to answer back, tended to have higher blood pressure.

Schedule an uninterrupted forty-minute block of time once a week in a comfortable, relaxed, quiet setting. One person speaks for twenty minutes while the other listens without responding. Then the roles are reversed. The object is to be able to talk freely about whatever you're thinking or feeling without worrying about judgment or criticism. Under the usual circumstances, if we express something that makes our partner uncomfortable, we get a negative reaction right away. With this exercise the listener will still react to the words or ideas that trigger discomfort, but will not be allowed to respond. The more the listener focuses on his or her own reaction, the less he or she is actually listening. The more you practice listening, the better you become at letting go of your own thoughts and feelings and at focusing on those of your partner. Some people have described this exercise as almost meditative, as it requires you to empty your mind of your own thoughts as you listen.

As the speaker, try not to dwell on the relating of current events, but concentrate more on the feelings these situations have elicited in you. If you're the second speaker, avoid a critique of what your partner just said. It is best not to comment on anything that was said during the exercise for up to three days following it. Creating a safe environment for expressing our feelings and allowing ourselves to be vulnerable with our spouses are extremely valuable tools for building trust, understanding, acceptance, and, at times, exhilarating feelings of intimacy. The last couple to whom we recommended this exercise said: "It felt wonderful to have his total attention," and "I really liked the fact that she was just listening without giving me any advice." This exercise is described in more detail in Maggie Scarf's book *Intimate Partners*.

A couple's ability to manage conflict is the best predictor of a successful marriage. Another helpful communication exercise, one that is highly effective for resolving conflict, is called "mirroring," or "reflective listening." This skill assists couples in slowing down the intensity of their interaction, and assures that that which is being communicated is accurately interpreted and validated. What is essential in this exercise is to *let go* of resolving the conflict, and instead to thoroughly focus on understanding each other's perspective. This is accomplished by paraphrasing short segments of conversation that consist of thoughts, and especially feelings, that are expressed without blame. In the book *Getting the Love You Want,* by Harville Hendrix, you can find an in-depth description of this technique.

The foundation of all communication exercises is to learn to let go of the need to be right. Your feelings are always the "right" ones. Couples are amazed by the information they get when they really listen to each other, and how this heightened awareness helps to resolve conflict. What is most important is that you don't attempt to convince your partner to do things your way, but for each of you to understand, appreciate, and respect one another's differences.

This level of communication will help to create not only greater intimacy but better health as well. That's the finding of Ohio State University researcher Janice Kiecolt-Glaser, who studied ninety newlywed couples as they discussed difficult issues —from money to in-laws—during videotaped sessions. By comparing before-and-after blood samples, researchers found that partners who resorted to hostile tactics showed measurably greater drops in immune function than did husbands and wives who took a more supportive, less adversarial position.

Requests

When you commit to each other, you enter into a relationship in which you have promised to give and receive love. Since each of us is different, what feels like love to one person might not even be noticed by another. Most of us attempt to love our partners in ways that feel like love to us, and are surprised when they do not react as we would. A good method of eliminating this problem is simply to tell each other what feels good. To ensure that you receive more of what you want, write three requests of your spouse. These should consist of actions or behaviors that you, the requester, perceive as most loving. Like the affirmations, the requests should contain only positive directions and should be as specific as possible. Some examples might be: I would like you to give me two hugs daily; I would like you to spend one afternoon each week with me; I would like you to buy me flowers once a week; I would like you to cook dinner once a week. It can be quite a revelation when someone you have lived with for many years, a person whom you thought you knew well, tells you what they *really* need from you. This exercise helps explain your own feelings of betrayal when your loving actions were not reciprocated. We often expect our partners to be mind readers: "He should have known what I wanted"; "She ought to have been able to tell how I felt." We really can't know exactly unless we are told. Be specific, make requests, and get what you need. It is extremely important to thank your partner for complying with any request. The requested task might not have been an easy or natural thing for him or her to do—otherwise you wouldn't have had to ask in the first place. Acknowledge the effort and even greater compliance will follow.

Having Fun Together

The pressures and responsibilities of daily life in America make it difficult to remember to have fun. For many couples, the glue that reinforces their relationship is the memory of enjoyment they shared during their courtship and early years together. To rekindle some of that earlier excitement and sweep away the cobwebs of routine and boredom, it helps to schedule fun activities together regularly. Plan a day or half-day each week to spend together away from home in an activity one of you has chosen. Alternate the responsibility for the choice of activity. Being out of the house, unaccompanied by friends or other family members, can help you focus attention on each other. Although it is more difficult, it is also possible, even with young children, to plan an enjoyable and perhaps an exciting evening at home, after the kids are in bed. Choosing something neither of you has ever tried before can add a sense of adventure to your play. If you can manage it, plan one weekend a month out of town. You might be surprised at how refreshing and invigorating regularly scheduled short trips can be for your relationship. These two-day excursions might be just what you need, especially if a real vacation isn't feasible.

Eye Gazing

Similar to "Eye Contact," which I mentioned in Chapter 12, this exercise is described in *The Art of Sexual Ecstasy,* by Margo Anand. It can be practiced for five minutes with your partner as frequently as you'd like. The directions are very simple:

1. Sit facing each other, either in chairs or cross-legged on the floor or kneeling. (If you are on the floor, sit on a thick pillow to keep your spine straight while your back is relaxed.)
2. Touch each other in a way that feels relaxing, such as lightly holding hands.
3. Close your eyes, breathe deeply and slowly. Pay attention to your body and how it feels—any tightness or discomfort; just notice but do nothing about it. Check in with your feelings —happy, sad, worried, etc. Again just notice and accept them. Notice the thoughts in your mind. Are there any judgments about you or your partner? Let them just pass.
4. When you feel quiet, send a little signal to your partner— such as a gentle squeeze of the hand—and wait for the return

signal. Open your eyes and allow your gaze to connect with that of your partner. Keeping your eyes relaxed, look into the left eye of your partner.

5. Allow yourself to be drawn completely into the present moment. Stay connected while staying aware of your breathing, centered in yourself.

6. Say silently to yourselves, "You love me" or "We are one" or any meaningful words of connection. As you repeat this to yourself, feel open to receiving your partner's love and appreciation. Let your eyes be windows to your soul. Allow yourself to *receive* your partner's love.

7. Recognize the essential humanness in your partner that is equally present in yourself. Simply be—have no particular goal except experiencing yourselves moment to moment.

8. Notice the rhythm of your breath and that of your partner. Without effort, see if you can gradually harmonize your breathing until you are inhaling and exhaling together. Let the breathing be simple and subtle.

Parenting

Don't expect any quick fix or magic cures in this section. A magician I'm not—just another parent trying to do my best. I have no simple approaches to what many see as life's most challenging full-time job. However, we can also choose to look at parenting as one of life's most enriching experiences—as a chance to play, to feel more in touch with our own "inner child"—and to let go of ourselves and experience selflessness. In dealing with teenagers, in particular, we are provided with a wonderful vehicle for practicing forgiveness, unconditional love, trust, self-acceptance, self-awareness, and most of all, patience.

A useful guideline in the process of learning effective parenting might be to ask yourself regularly, "Will this (action, response, activity, or demand) of mine help my child's self-esteem?" The same principle holds true in parenting as it does in marriage: *To love another is to help that person better love himself or herself.* Obviously, as human beings, we are not always able to meet this ideal. Children are constantly trying to expand their limits and are testing ours at the same time. While they seek greater independence, our job is to balance our own degree of comfort—which includes our values and levels of fear, faith, and trust—with what will most benefit these young explorers for whom we are responsible. It requires a great deal of awareness to appreciate who these unique persons are and to know how best to provide them the safety and base of security they need in order to develop their independence and discover their hidden talents and gifts. Most of us take great pride in our children's achievements and strengths and disavow any connection to their flaws. Still, our children are composites of genetic inheritance from both parents, environmental influences, and the intangible factor of their own unique spirit. This combination produces a human being altogether different from any other. As parents we must respect and acknowledge this difference, even though at times we feel as if our children are extensions of ourselves. What we have considered to be good or bad for us might be just the opposite for our children.

In the field of family therapy, the family is usually seen from the "systems" approach. This view holds that if a member's behavior is harmful to himself or others, the problem and the solution lie not solely within that individual but in the entire family system. This perspective encourages parents to look at their roles and the partial responsibility they share for the problem. A child's crisis can be a mirror reflecting to a parent an imbalance in his or her own individual system as well as in the family system. One of the significant advantages of family therapy is that change often occurs more rapidly than in individual psychotherapy. In much the same way that holistic medicine refrains from treating the physical symptom without looking at the entire person, the systems approach recognizes the need for family therapy when one member of the family is suffering. If this is a situation that applies to your family, I strongly recommend family counseling.

I have mentioned that anger is a primary cause of sinus disease. The focus of that anger is often either yourself, your spouse, or your children. Now that you know several ways to release it, there is another way to use anger beneficially, particularly with regard to your children. I have found consistently that the aspects of a child's behavior that most upset a parent are those the parent likes least about him- or herself. I guess it's just easier to be angry with our kids than with ourselves. These disturbing behavior patterns become most apparent during adolescence, which merely adds to the challenge of parenting teenagers. For instance, suppose you believe your child has innate ability in a certain sport, with a musical instrument, or in a creative art, but the child refuses to pursue it for fear of making mistakes or looking awkward or silly as a beginner, or perhaps for no reason at all. You feel a very strong reaction, become furious, and find yourself insisting that the youngster at least *try* this new endeavor. Whenever you react so strongly, it's time to stop, reflect, and use the situation as a mirror. Perhaps this particular incident is reminiscent of your own fear of trying new things. It might be bringing up feelings of frustration and anger with yourself for the many times you failed to realize your own potential. Out of your anger with the child can arise a chance for you to see yourself more clearly and to forgive and accept both yourself and the child. Opportunities for loving often present themselves in unusual ways.

Good parenting requires both time and consistency. If you've completed a personal vision list and a shared vision list with your partner, they might provide a good idea of which values you would like to instill in your children. These values can serve as a guide for the rules you both implement and consistently adhere to as parents. Setting limits is just another way of loving your child and yourself.

Time seems to be the ingredient most lacking in today's society. In the "typical" American family both parents are employed outside the home, and the most striking change for this generation of teenagers is their isolation. A high percentage of these children have been with many different caretakers, often spending more hours with them than with their own parents. For these and many other reasons, this is not an easy period in which to be growing up in the United States. No one is even certain what the normal or typical American family looks like. From the 1990 Census, we've learned that 50 percent of all children in the nation under eighteen live in a "traditional nuclear family," while the other 50 percent live "with a stepparent and step-siblings, in a single-parent household, with other relatives or non-relatives or in some other arrangement." Although a new norm is being created, nearly 73 percent of all American children do live with married parents. But even in the single-parent and two-career households, if the commitment is there, time for the family can be found. Family dinners, for instance, when every-one eats together, don't have to be a lost tradition. I suggest trying to share at least this one daily meal as a chance to converse and get to know one another. Make sure the television is off. The average American watches about thirty hours of television a week, which must mean that it has become both a distraction from and a frequent guest at dinner tables across the country. A recent Gallup poll revealed that among those who dine at home in the company of others, nearly four out of ten watch TV, study, work, or read while eating.

Other ways to spend time as a family are to worship together each week at church or synagogue and to designate a regularly scheduled time during the weekend for a fun activity. You can rotate the leader, so that each family member has a chance to choose the activity. The value of play cannot be overemphasized. Having fun together can sometimes accomplish what many ses-sions of family therapy are unable to do.

What parents really need to do is show that their love is un-conditional, that nothing a child does or fails to do will diminish that love, and that children do not have the power to make or break their parents emotionally by their actions or achievements. That's really all there is to it! Isn't that simple?

ALTRUISM

The late Hans Selye, a pioneer in modern stress research, thought that by helping people you inspire their gratitude and affection, and that the warmth that results somehow protects you from stress. More recent studies suggest that this warm feeling might well come from endorphins—the brain's natural producers of euphoria. Even watching others help a third party seems to help the observer. In a striking study at Harvard University, psychologist David McClelland showed students a film of Mother Teresa, the embodiment of altruism, working among Calcutta's sick and poor. Analyses of the students' saliva revealed an increase in immunoglobulin A, an antibody that can combat respiratory infections. Even the students who consciously had no sympathy for Mother Teresa responded with enhanced immunity. Epidemiologist James House and his colleagues at the University of Michigan's Survey Research Center studied more than 2,700 men in Tecumseh, Michigan, for almost fourteen years to see how social relationships affected mortality rates. Those who did regular volunteer work had death rates two and one-half times lower than those who didn't.

The evidence is mounting that selflessness not only feels good but is healthy. When we freely choose to care, we seem to get as much, or more, than we give. However, as Ornstein and Sobel point out in *Healthy Pleasures,* being in control and having a choice are crucial to the health benefits of giving. Those who must care for sick loved ones for long periods often report more, not less, stress and illness.

The closer our contact with those we help, the greater the benefits seem to be. By far my greatest rewards as a physician have come from the gratitude and appreciation I've felt from so many of my patients. Most of us need to feel that we matter to someone, but you needn't be in the healing arts to derive that pleasure. There is a growing number of needy people in our society—homeless, hungry, parentless, and illiterate—and there are many ways to help them.

Destructive self-centeredness can be treated with a healthy dose of selflessness. But the treatment works best if your generosity comes from the heart and is not calculated to benefit you. In *Healthy Pleasures,* Ornstein and Sobel devote a chapter to "selfless pleasures." They close with the following:

Healthy altruism comes from the understanding that you and those around you are part of the same human community or social body. When one person suffers or is deprived, all of us are affected. It is for this reason that religions counsel generosity and service to others. The human community is strengthened and the server, too, benefits.

It is important, even vital, to be able to connect with other people and to be part of life in general; our lives, our health, and our destiny are connected with that of others. The great surprise of human evolution may be that the highest form of selfishness is selflessness.

SOCIAL HEALTH RECOMMENDATIONS: A SUMMARY

- Social health is defined by our degree of *connection to other human beings*. American culture has bred a society suffering from isolation, alienation, aloneness, and hostility.
- *Support groups* are small groups of people who meet regularly to share views on common ailments, problems, values, or beliefs, or for the purpose of enhancing spiritual growth. Anyone with a chronic disease or who feels a lack of community should consider either joining or forming a group.
- *Marriage* is a spiritual practice of learning to love your "neighbor" as yourself, balancing independence and intimacy. Some helpful exercises include sharing a vision listing common goals for the relationship; listening (one partner speaks for twenty minutes while the spouse listens without any response, then the reverse) making three requests of your spouse for actions or things that would make you feel loved; having fun together regularly scheduling a block of time for enjoying each other's company; and eye gazing.
- *Parenting* is a challenging opportunity to practice unconditional love on our children as well as ourselves. It requires a

balance between teaching independence and allowing the exploration of potential gifts and setting comfortable limits. It takes consistency, time, and the recognition of your child's uniqueness. Try to define your values and establish rules in accordance with them; create time for family dinners and family fun. Parenting might be life's most difficult and most rewarding full-time job.

- *Altruism*—helping others—can be pleasurable as well as provide a boost to the immune system. Healthy selflessness can be an antidote for the negative effects of self-involvement. Helping others with genuine goodwill brings a powerful feeling of connection, a sense of unity, and the recognition that in giving to others you are ultimately giving to yourself.

Chapter 14

A GUIDE TO HOLISTIC SPECIALTIES

W hat I have presented in chapters 6 through 13 is an intro-
duction to and overview of holistic medicine and holistic
health. The material was meant to provide you with some idea of
the breadth of this field and to give you enough information to
begin to practice it on yourself. Conveying the full scope of this
healing art would require an encyclopedic text.

As a general practitioner of holistic medicine, just as I did as a
general practitioner of conventional medicine, I serve as a "jack
of all trades," with a working knowledge of each component of
holistic health. However, just as there are many medical specialties, there are also many holistic specialties. Most medical specialties focus on one part or system of the body; for example, ear,
nose, and throat specialists work only on the neck and above,
including the sinuses. Holistic specialties, on the other hand,
might encompass all parts of the body but might be limited in the
degree to which they address the various aspects of holistic
health. Some holistic specialists focus almost solely on the physical, others on the mental or emotional. There are those who
work almost exclusively on spiritual or social health. One common denominator with almost every one of these healing arts
and disciplines is that medical science has not recognized their
therapeutic value, and therefore they have been largely ignored
—even scorned—by many in the allopathic medical community.

In honoring its commitments to heal and to teach, holistic medicine encourages an openness to complementary concepts as well as an understanding that what is not scientifically proven is not necessarily invalid.

The four holistic specialties that I will discuss briefly in this chapter are all, like allopathic medicine, physically oriented. However, they are all based, at least in part, on a holistic philosophy that recognizes the integration of body, mind, and spirit in the creation of health. They are osteopathic medicine, naturopathic medicine, Oriental or Traditional Chinese medicine, and homeopathic medicine. I have chosen these four because I have had a great deal of personal experience with each one and know that all of them can be effective in treating each of the chronic respiratory diseases. For the same reason, I have included a short discussion of reflexology at the end of the chapter.

OSTEOPATHIC MEDICINE

The field of medicine with which I am most familiar is the one in which I received my formal training. Osteopathic medicine is, not coincidentally, the predecessor of holistic medicine. In theory and philosophy *it is holistic medicine,* but in practice it usually is not as comprehensive an approach. Although we were taught a different perspective, many osteopathic physicians today are practicing medicine very similarly to our allopathic brethren, relying heavily on pharmaceutical drugs and surgical treatment.

In 1968, on my first day as an osteopathic medical student, I learned the basic philosophy of osteopathy, called "The Totality of Man." I was taught that in my first encounter with a sick patient, I was to focus on the person with the disease, and not the other way around. This concept further instructed that, when initially evaluating a patient to determine the diagnosis, essential to that patient's history are the emotional, social, and spiritual aspects of his or her life, i.e., "the total person." My initial reaction was one of "So what's the big deal? This just sounds like good common sense. Any thorough and caring doctor would look at the whole person in attempting to understand his or her disease process, right?" I was wrong. Although my father was an M.D. radiologist, who spent almost all of his professional life immersed in the high-tech world of X-rays, I hadn't realized that allopathic medical training was entirely focused on the science of medicine and the diagnosis and treatment of disease and its symptoms. The study of the mind was still in its infancy and was relegated to a secondary status with little or no connection to physical disease. The art of healing and the concept of health as a condition of wholeness were missing. Needless to say, the word "spirit" was never mentioned in allopathic classrooms as a part of the curriculum. Osteopathy also teaches an appreciation of the body's ability to heal itself.

Unbeknownst to me at the time, I had arrived at just the right place to begin my medical training. I was learning preventive medicine, holistic health, and to treat the whole person while diagnosing and treating the disease. Since my educational objective was to become a family doctor, it seemed to be a perfect philosophical fit. The fact that the vast majority of osteopathic graduates became family physicians was additional confirmation that I had made the right choice. At the time, less than 2 percent of allopathic medical students entered family medicine.

Not surprisingly, osteopathic medicine was founded by an M.D., in 1874. Andrew Taylor Still was a fourth-generation M.D. who, after losing four of his own children one winter to an epidemic of meningitis, began to question the completeness of his medical training. He also suffered from terrible headaches for which he had found no solution in the medical model of his day.

In the truly Hippocratic tradition, he became a seeker of answers to his own challenging medical problem. He most likely grave-robbed in order to study anatomy, since this was not a part of traditional medical training at that time. Combining what he learned from studying anatomy with what he already knew about physiology and neurology, he solved his own chronic headaches using a makeshift "hands-on" approach, by stringing a rope between two trees and lying with the base of his skull on the rope until his headache went away. He became widely known for his effective, noninvasive, hands-on approach, and was referred to as a "bone-setter." Dr. Still was unsuccessful in his attempts to have his ideas and methods incorporated into the traditional medical model. Since his apprentices (seven-year apprenticeships were the accepted method of medical training in his day) were being taught medical "heresy," they were not granted the traditional M.D. degree. Instead, they were called D.O.s—Doctors of Osteopathy. (The Latin root *osteo* means "bone," and *patheia* is Greek for "passion" or "suffering.")

When medical schools opened around the turn of the century, osteopathic students were still thought to be medical heretics, and thus began the two different forms of complete medical training, with two separate medical degrees—M.D. and D.O. Today, osteopathic medical schools have a very similar four-year curriculum to allopathic schools, with most of the same courses and textbooks but two very basic differences: *osteopathic medical schools teach the holistic philosophy and the hands-on approach to diagnosis and treatment, called Osteopathic Manipulative Treatment (OMT),* based upon the interrelationship of structure and function. There have been several attempts made by M.D.s to amalgamate the two medical professions, but D.O.s have steadfastly refused to relinquish their unique identity and their approach to health care.

It is unfortunate that the majority of osteopathic physicians today have not maintained the original philosophy of their profession, and their practice of medicine differs very little from that of their M.D. colleagues. However, as a minority professional group, with far less public recognition than M.D.s, it is easy to understand why so many D.O.s have relinquished their identity and become professionally assimilated. My own medical career is a good example. After graduating from the Philadelphia College of Osteopathic Medicine, I trained in a three-year family practice residency at Mercy Medical Center in Denver. It was an excellent program, but at the time I was the only D.O. in the residency program and in the entire hospital. It was very difficult to maintain a separate identity. It wasn't until I joined the American Holistic Medical Association in 1988 that I reconnected with my osteopathic heritage.

Andrew Taylor Still never intended to start a separate school of medicine. Yet today there are sixteen colleges of osteopathic medicine and more than 36,000 osteopathic physicians practicing in the United States. They represent every medical and surgical specialty. Dr. Still's contributions to health care are particularly important to note today as holistic medicine finally emerges from the 120-year-old cocoon of osteopathic medicine. During the late nineteenth century, he did the following:

- Founded and dedicated the science of osteopathic medicine to the search for holistic health care principles, treatment, and therapies.
- Believed that physicians should study prevention as well as cure, and treat "patients"—not "symptoms."
- Was among the first to identify the human immune system and develop a system for stimulating it naturally.
- Believed that the human body is in nature and function designed to operate as a perfect, harmonious whole, and that disease in one part affects all other parts.
- Predicted that this country would become a nation of drug addicts and alcoholics within the century if physicians continued to overprescribe addictive drugs.
- Believed that the most important drugs and the ones most worthy of study are those produced within the human body.
- Warned that women were far too often the victims of needless surgeries.
- Was the first to welcome women and minorities into medical school.

As we approach the twenty-first century, the contributions made by Dr. Still and osteopathic medicine to health care are enjoying much greater recognition and respect from both the public and the medical community. As for the treatment of the common chronic respiratory conditions, OMT in the hands of a skilled osteopathic physician can be quite helpful for all four of these ailments. There are five primary forms of OMT techniques: ligaments/fascia (soft tissue), cranial, high velocity/low amplitude, strain/counterstrain, and muscle energy. For the head, nose, sinuses, and lungs, I am familiar with significant benefits from all but the latter two techniques. I have been especially impressed with cranial therapy for chronic sinusitis. Although this is almost always performed by the physician, I've recently learned about a cranial technique originated by John Upledger, D.O., one of the leading teachers of cranial osteopathy in the United States. He recommends inserting two racquet balls into a sock, tying a knot at the open end of the sock, placing the balls under the base of the skull (it's actually the occiput—the most prominent point in the back of your head), and resting the head on them for fifteen to thirty minutes a day. This procedure allows the sinuses to drain and relieves nasal congestion. A *Sinus Survival* reader in Seattle who regularly uses this technique reported to me that it is more effective than any decongestant she's ever tried and has no unpleasant side effects.

Other OMT techniques, such as fascial release and lymphatic drainage when performed around the ribs and sternum, can be quite helpful in the treatment of asthma and bronchitis.

Although it's not always the case, in general if you are looking for a more holistic primary care physician, I would choose a D.O.

NATUROPATHIC MEDICINE

Naturopathic physicians (N.D.s) are specialists in natural medicine. They are trained at four-year naturopathic medical colleges and are educated in the conventional medical sciences. They treat both acute and chronic disease, and their treatments are drawn from clinical nutrition, herbal or botanical medicine, homeopathy, Traditional Chinese medicine, physical medicine, exercise therapy, counseling, acupuncture, and hydrotherapy. Some naturopaths might combine several or all of these therapies, whereas others might specialize in one specific area.

The basic principles of naturopathy are based on the concept that the body is a self-healing organism. The naturopathic physician enhances the body's own natural immune response through noninvasive measures and health promotion. Rather than treat the symptoms, naturopaths strive to uncover the underlying cause of patients' diseases, looking at physical, mental, and emotional factors. Health is seen not as the absence of symptoms, but as the absence of the causes of symptoms. Prevention and wellness are vital principles in naturopathy. These physicians are trained to know which patients they can treat safely and which ones they need to refer to other health care practitioners. As teachers, naturopaths facilitate the growth of patients' responsibility for their own health and spark the enthusiasm and motivation patients need to make fundamental lifestyle changes. The origins of naturopathic philosophy extend as far back as Hippocrates, who set forth the principles "Do no harm" and "Let your food be your medicine, and your medicine be your food."

As a distinct American health care profession, naturopathic medicine is almost 100 years old. Early in this century there were more than twenty naturopathic medical colleges. Today there are only two—in Portland, Oregon, and Seattle, Washington. In the 1940s and 1950s, with the advent of more technological medicine, the increased popularity of pharmaceutical drugs, and the belief that such drugs could eliminate all disease, naturopathy experienced a decline. During the past two decades, however, as more people have begun to seek alternatives to conventional medicine, it has seen a resurgence in popularity.

Naturopathy seems to be making its greatest contributions to the healing arts in the fields of immunology, clinical nutrition, and botanical medicine. Much of the vitamin and herbal regimen for the treatment of sinusitis and the strengthening of the immune system described in chapter 8 comes from naturopathic medicine.

TRADITIONAL CHINESE MEDICINE

Traditional Chinese medicine is the primary health care system currently used by approximately 30 percent of the world's population. It is believed to be one of the oldest medical systems in existence, dating back almost 5,000 years. The practice of acupuncture (a method of using fine needles to stimulate invisible lines of energy running beneath the surface of the skin) is the component of Chinese medicine most familiar to Americans, but the system also includes Chinese herbology, moxabustion (the burning of an herb at acupuncture points), massage, diet, exercise, and meditation.

In ancient China, doctors were not paid if patients under their care became sick. The job of the physician was to keep patients healthy. Chinese medicine believes that a certain process happens before the body develops a problem or disease. A Chinese medicine practitioner (O.M.D., Doctor of Oriental Medicine) looks for this process or pattern of disharmony. Through questioning, observation, and palpation, a practitioner can determine a person's current state of health and the problems that individual will be at highest risk for developing in the future. In this way, Chinese medicine is an effective preventive therapy.

Traditional Chinese medicine is based on a history, philosophy, and sociology very different from those of the West. Over thousands of years it has developed a unique understanding of how the body works. Practitioners of Chinese medicine see disease as an imbalance between the body's nutritive substances, called yin, and the functional activity of the body, called yang. This imbalance causes a disruption of the flow of vital energy that circulates through pathways in the body known as meridians. This vital energy, called qi or chi, keeps the blood circulating, warms the body, and fights disease. The intimate connection between the organ systems of the body and the meridians enables the practice of acupuncture to intercede and rebalance the body's energy through stimulation of specific points along the meridians.

People who have used Chinese medicine for a particular physical symptom frequently experience improvement in seemingly unrelated problems. This occurs because the Chinese approach tends to restore the body to a greater degree of balance, thereby enhancing its capacity for self-healing. The entire person is treated, not just the symptom, and the relationship of body, mind, emotions, spirit, and environment are all taken into account.

The World Health Organization has published a list of over fifty diseases successfully treated with acupuncture. Included on the list are sinusitis, asthma, arthritis, the common cold, headaches (including migraine), constipation, diarrhea, sciatica, and lower back pain. Acupuncture has also been effective in the treatment of allergies, addictions, insomnia, stress, depression, infertility, and menstrual problems.

Chinese herbs are the most common element of Chinese medicine as it is currently practiced in China. The herbs are becoming more popular in the United States, but it is still much easier to find a licensed acupuncturist (L.Ac., C.A., R.Ac., Dipl. Ac.) than an O.M.D. who is knowledgeable about Chinese herbs as well as acupuncture. Beginning in April 1995, there will be national board certification in Chinese herbal medicine, offering the degree Dipl. C.H. As more schools of Traditional Chinese medicine are established in this country, these licensed practitioners will be much easier to find.

Pharmaceutical drugs are usually made by synthetically producing the active ingredient of an herb. Medicinal plants differ from the isolated active ingredients in synthetic drugs because they contain associate substances that balance the medicinal effects. Uncomfortable side effects are generally the result of the removal of these associate substances. Chinese herbs are capable of regenerating, vitalizing, and balancing the vital energy, tissue, and organs of the body without harmful side effects. They can be taken in pill or powder form or as raw herbs made into tea.

Sinusitis, allergies, asthma, and bronchitis can all be treated effectively with a combination of acupuncture and Chinese herbs. The herbs most commonly used for sinuses and allergies are: Bi Yan Pian, Pe Min Kan Wan, Seven Forests-Xanthium 12, and Pollen Allergy. Acute bronchitis can be treated symptomatically during an attack according to the color and consistency of the mucus. If it is profuse, clear, or white, use one of the following: Er Chen Wan, Chi Kuan Yen Wan, or Hsiao Ke Chuan. If the mucus is thick and yellow, the recommended herbs are: Ching Fei Yi Huo Pien, Jie Geng Wan, or Pinellia Expectorant Pills.

Although all four of these conditions are commonly treated with Chinese medicine, only sinusitis and bronchitis lend themselves to self-treatment with herbs. Allergies and especially asthma are considered to be complex problems and should be treated by a qualified practitioner of Traditional Chinese medicine, who can not only treat the acute attacks but also prevent flare-ups from occurring in between these crises.

Acupressure works according to the same principle as acupuncture, using the same points on the meridians, but with direct finger pressure used in place of needles to stimulate these points. Of the two techniques, acupuncture is generally more effective, but acupressure allows you to do it yourself. The two diagrams in Figure 14-1. illustrate the acupressure points you can use for sinusitis. Pressure should be applied gently with your index fingers; abrupt application detracts from the relaxing effects. According to Cathryn Bauer in her book *Acupressure for Everybody,* there are a few basic principles concerning how to press points sensitively.

1.   Your hands should be clean, warm, and dry. Start by holding your palm over the point for a moment. Then, using the tip of your index finger, probe the area gently until you feel a slight dip; this is the acupressure point.

2.   Press in lightly, holding your finger in this position until you feel the muscle relax. Increase the pressure very slowly. Stop pressing when you feel that you're forcing it; just hold the pressure steady. Pay close attention to the way the point feels. Acupressure points often become warm as muscle tension eases.

3.   Keep the pressure steady until the point is neither warm nor cool and pulses steadily. (The pulsation is not as strong as the pulse in your wrists and neck.) This usually takes at least three minutes, and it may take ten minutes or longer to release tensions if your symptoms are acute.

4.   When the pulse is throbbing evenly, ease your fingertip off the point. An abrupt release can feel unpleasant.

Points 1, 2, and 3 are helpful for anyone with a sinus condition. Points 4 through 8 need only be used if those places are sore to the touch (using mild pressure). Stimulating these acupressure points can help to relieve sinus pain and congestion, as well as the symptoms of nasal allergy. Keep in mind that symptom relief may not occur for up to thirty minutes. The points shown in Figure 14-1 are defined and described in the following material.

1. LI (large intestine) 4—in the webbing between thumb and index finger. To locate the exact point, place your thumb beside your index finger; the hump, or "meatiest" part, of the web is the spot. Stimulate both hands. This point addresses problems anywhere in your head, such as a headache, toothache, or eye or vision problem.

2. Extra bitong—along the edge of the nasal bone in the groove along the nose.

3. LI 20—beside the nose at the midpoint of its widest part.

4. ST (stomach) 2—in the tiny notch on the bony ridge below the eye, in line with the pupil.

5. UB (urinary bladder) 2—on the nasal end of the eyebrow in a small notch in the underlying bone.

6. Extra yin tang—midway between the nasal ends of the eyebrows.

7. Extra tai yang—in the depression of the temple (also a good point to use for headaches).

8. Extra yu yao—the middle of the eyebrow, in line with the pupil.

9. Along both sides of the bridge of the nose in the nasal corner of the eye socket. This is not an official Chinese acupressure point, but many sinus patients have obtained relief using it.

Acute attacks of asthma and bronchitis can be helped by applying acupressure to a point on the anterior midline (over your breastbone) midway between the nipples. This point is called Tanzhong.

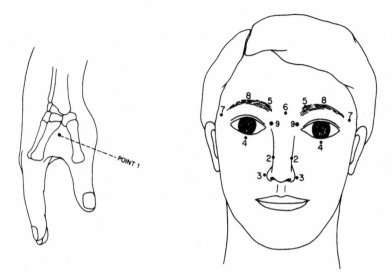

FIGURE 14-1. *Finger Acupressure*

HOMEOPATHIC MEDICINE

Homeopathy is a form of treatment that gently nudges the body toward a healthier state. Its practice was begun in 1820 by Samuel Hahnemann, a German physician, who believed that whatever caused disease would also cure it. The Latin phrase *similia similibus curantur* (like shall be cured by like) is the cornerstone of homeopathic medicine. According to Hahnemann, the proper remedy for an illness that exhibits any set of symptoms in a sick person is that substance that would produce the same set of symptoms in a healthy person. This "law of similars" was not original with Hahnemann. The idea had been advanced by philosophers and physicians for thousands of years, and Hahnemann acknowledged his debt to Hippocrates, in whose writings the principle of "like cures like" appears. Hahnemann, however, was the first to build a consistent system based on this principle.

Homeopathy flourished in the 1800s and hasn't changed much since then. The Hahnemann School of Medicine in Philadelphia was originally a school of homeopathic medicine. The advent of rigorous scientific medicine in the United States during this century almost completely eliminated homeopathy. Today, this healing discipline is once again on the rise all over the world, including this country. The National Center for Homeopathic Medicine in Washington, D.C., estimates that there are somewhere between one and two thousand practitioners in the United States and that about 300 of them are M.D.'s or D.O.'s. Homeopathy has fared much better in other parts of the world. One-third of all French physicians practice it. In Britain, members of the royal family have been cared for by homeopathic physicians since the reign of Queen Victoria. Homeopathy is taught and used in hospitals and physicians' offices in Scotland, Germany, Austria, Switzerland, India, Mexico, Chile, Brazil, and Argentina.

Homeopathy uses infinitesimal or microdoses of natural materials—that is, mineral, plant, or animal. Some standard homeopathic solutions might be as weak as one part in a hundred thousand. These mixtures must be shaken vigorously (succussed) in a carefully prescribed manner in order to be activated. Only tiny amounts of a substance are used, but homeopaths believe that the treatment works because even if the substance were reduced to a single molecule, or lost altogether, its "pattern" would remain in the liquid and could produce an effect. Scientific support for this theory was contained in a 1988 issue of the prestigious British journal *Nature*. The publication described a study from a French laboratory headed by a well-known medical research scientist in the fields of allergy and immunology. The research team demonstrated that a solution that had contained a human antibody, yet was so diluted that not a molecule of it was left, had produced a response in human blood cells. Science cannot explain precisely how this could happen, but the reasons why many pharmaceutical drugs, including aspirin, are effective are also still largely a mystery.

Homeopathic medicines are not required to meet the safe and

effective standards of the Food and Drug Administration. They are sold by mail, in drugstores, and in health-food stores. Most are nonprescription and legally can be advertised as remedies only for self-limiting conditions, such as colds. Prescription homeopathic substances can be dispensed only by someone licensed to prescribe drugs.

Many patients who seek the care of a homeopathic practitioner have a chronic condition considered incurable by conventional medicine. An effective homeopathic treatment for sinusitis is kali bichromium at 30c every hour for four or five doses. A homeopathic nasal spray that works quite well is called Euphorbium Nasal Spray, which is manufactured in Germany and distributed by Biological Homeopathic Industries in Albuquerque, New Mexico. A double-blind study published in the journal *Biological Therapy* in January 1995 showed Euphorbium to be effective in relieving the symptoms of nasal congestion and headaches in people with chronic sinusitis. The study took place over a five-month period, during which time the patients were instructed to spray twice in each nostril four times a day. One-half of the group were using a placebo. This product can be found in many health food stores.

REFLEXOLOGY

I do not regard reflexology as a holistic specialty, but I have included it here because of its similarity to acupressure and because it can be an effective complement in treating chronic respiratory disease. Reflexology is an art and science that makes use of the reflex areas in the feet and hands that correspond to all of the glands, organs, and parts of the body. It employs a unique method of using the thumb and fingers on the reflex areas to relieve stress and tension, improve blood supply and promote the unblocking of nerve impulses, and help the body achieve homeostasis—a state of balance. Reflexology is a natural, noninvasive therapy that grew out of the theories and techniques of acupuncture and acupressure. From hieroglyphic paintings found on a wall in an ancient Egyptian tomb, there is strong evidence to suggest that reflexology was practiced before 2330 B.C. From other ancient texts, illustrations, and artifacts, it is known that the early Japanese, Indians, and Russians, as well as the Chinese and Egyptians, worked on the feet to promote good health.

However, as with Chinese medicine, it was not until the twentieth century that reflexology gained acceptance in the Western world. Foot reflexology was introduced in the United States in 1913 by William H. Fitzgerald, M.D., following his discovery of the Chinese method of zone therapy. While serving as the head of the Nose and Throat Department of St. Francis Hospital in Hartford, Connecticut, he developed the modern zone theory of the human body, arguing that some parts of the body correspond to other parts and offering as proof the fact that applying pressure to one area anesthetizes a corresponding area.

In the 1930s, Eunice Ingham, a physiotherapist for Joseph S. Riley, M.D., another pioneer in the field of zone therapy, found the feet to be the most responsive areas for working the zones because they were extremely sensitive. Eventually she "mapped" all of the points on the feet that corresponded with points in other parts of the body. She discovered that an alternating pressure applied with the thumb and fingers on the various points on the feet had therapeutic effects far beyond the limited use to which zone therapy had been previously employed, including the reduction of pain. Thus, reflexology was born.

As with acupuncture, reflexology attempts to strengthen and balance the intangible life energy, chi or qi, that flows in zones or meridians throughout the body. Reflexologists specify ten energy zones that run the length of the body from head to toe—five on each side of the body ending in each foot and running down the arms into the tips of the fingers. Not only do these zones run lengthwise, but they pass through the body; therefore, a zone located on the front of the body can also be reached from behind. All of the organs and parts of the body lie along one or more of these zones. Stimulating or working any zone in the foot by applying pressure with the thumbs and fingers affects the entire zone throughout the body. The actual physical mechanism that controls the ten zones in the body and feet is not fully under-stood, but it is a fact that reflexology is effective as an adjunct in the treatment of a variety of chronic ailments, probably as a result of its ability to induce deep states of relaxation. With this reduc-tion of stress in the body, there are many potential benefits. Circulation can be improved, toxins and waste products can be eliminated more easily, energy levels can be increased, and mental alertness, creativity, and productivity can be heightened.

I can attest personally to the state of relaxation that results from a reflexology session, and I have known patients suffering from chronic sinusitis who experienced dramatic relief through this treatment. Reflex therapy can be administered through alter-nating finger pressure or percussion. This can be applied using the fingers (usually the index finger, with a rotating method of compression massage) and thumb, or using percussion machines. Under my desk, I keep a device called a Reflex-Aid, a floor-mounted foot massage machine equipped with a spiked rubber ball. This allows me to massage the foot reflexes while I'm work-ing.

For anyone interested in trying this approach as a complement to their holistic health program, I recommend beginning with a visit to a reflexologist. See how it feels to have your feet worked on by a professional. Figure 14-2 illustrates the sinus points on the hands and the feet as well as the nose (allergies) and lung (asthma and bronchitis) points. Both hands have identical points in the webbing between the fingers. They can be stimulated with the thumb and index finger or even with the eraser of a pencil. Apply the pressure for twenty to thirty seconds and with enough force to cause some discomfort. The sinus points are the same on the soles of both feet. There are also three other points—liver and ileocecal valve (both on the right foot) and spleen (on the left)—that are important in treating the sinuses. Try stimulating all of these points on a daily basis and see what happens. If nothing else, you will be giving your feet, one of our most abused body parts, some welcome attention.

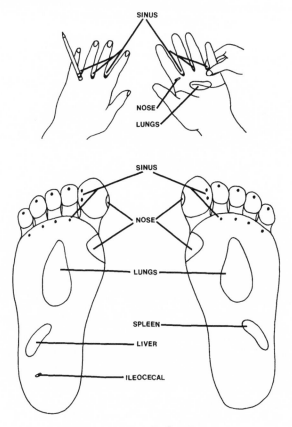

FIGURE 14-2. *Reflex Points*

Each of the holistic specialties offers a safe, noninvasive, and effective complement, and in some cases an alternative, to the conventional allopathic treatment of pharmaceutical drugs and surgery. Although they have the potential to significantly improve your condition, if your commitment is to *cure* your respiratory dis-ease—chronic sinusitis, allergies, asthma, or chronic bronchitis—you will still have to practice healing your mind and spirit as well as your body.

Chapter 15

THE TOP 10: READERS' MOST FREQUENTLY ASKED QUESTIONS

1. Where can I find a doctor who treats sinus problems the way you do?

Although you may not find someone who practices in exactly the same manner, a holistic physician will usually treat any chronic disease using an approach that is similar to the Sinus Survival Program. You can find a holistic physician in your area by writing to the American Holistic Medical Association, 4101 Lake Boone Trail, Suite 201, Raleigh, NC 27607, or calling (919) 787-5181 and requesting the Physician Referral Directory. The cost is $5, which includes shipping. Many members of this organization are familiar with *Sinus Survival,* and the program described in this book has become the "AHMA suggested" holistic medical treatment for chronic sinusitis.

2. Can you help me?

Yes, but it has to be done in person. Due to multiple professional commitments, I am able to see only a limited number of individuals in private consultation. Coming to see me is like going to school and taking an intensive course in self-healing. Your textbook is *Sinus Survival,* although there is other suggested reading that I've referred to in the book. Sessions last for about two hours and occur at monthly intervals. The basic Sinus Survival Program is taught in five sessions and parallels Part II of the book. The focus of the first consultation is on taking a complete holistic medical history and establishing a personalized physical and environmental health program. The second session deals with mental health, the third emotional health, the fourth social health, and fifth spiritual health. It is a course without exams or grades but with lots of homework. If you are interested in this personal program, I can be reached at (303) 978-1474.

For the past two years I have been teaching the Sinus Survival Program in a six-class course to groups of ten to twenty people. Classes are held every two or three weeks over a three-month period. The content is the same as the private consultations, and although the course isn't quite as personalized or as expensive, the results experienced by these students compare favorably to those of the individual patients whom I've seen.

Beginning in 1996, I'll be teaching sinus sufferers the entire Sinus Survival course in weekend workshops at the University of Colorado School of Medicine in conjunction with the Department of Otolaryngology. Together with the chairman of the department, Bruce Jafek, M.D., we have created the Nasal and Sinus Diseases Center. Prospective students for this course are jointly evaluated by Dr. Jafek and myself before beginning the workshops. Your progress and results will be well documented and contribute toward the scientific verification of the effectiveness of the Sinus Survival Program. This is a necessary but exciting step in the evolution of the program, and will eventually make medical insurance coverage possible for this nonsurgical treatment.

If you are interested in the Sinus Survival group course, contact the Department of Otolaryngology (Ear, Nose, and Throat) at (303) 270-7988 for registration information.

3. Where are the healthiest places to live in the United States with respect to air quality?
In Chapter 2 I've listed the most unhealthy cities according to the EPA with respect to specific air pollutants. However, there aren't any cities that I'm aware of—large or moderate-sized (more than 500,000 people)—that are not plagued by some de-

gree of air pollution. Living in a rural area (well beyond the suburbs of any large city) is almost always better than living in or near a city. Exceptions to this rule would include: heavy agricultural areas where there might be significant amounts of fertilizers, pesticides, and pollen polluting the air; proximity to or being downwind of a power plant, chemical plant, a major highway, or an airport; or any rural area that's downwind of a city and directly in the path of prevailing daily or seasonal wind patterns. The healthiest rural areas in the United States can be found along the West Coast (outside the coastal cities), along the Gulf Coast (except Texas), and the west coast of Florida.

If you want to live in or near a large city, the suburbs of the West Coast cities of Seattle, Portland, San Francisco, and San Diego, as well as Tampa and Miami, are probably the healthiest areas. Be sure to investigate through the Department of Health which suburban areas are better than others. If you can't move away from your present city, it would be a good idea to check with your local health department to find the least polluted suburb. Be especially concerned about high particulate levels as well as ozone and carbon monoxide.

4. What are the best furnace filters, air cleaners, and negative-ion generators?
See Chapter 7 and the "Product Index" for a complete rundown on recommended products.

5. What "Sinus Survival Products" are available?
A negative-ion generator called Sinus Survival Air Vitalizer is the most energy efficient and effective air cleaner I've found. It has been tested extensively in reputable laboratories and performs as well as the best HEPA air cleaners and at one-half to one-third the price. This ionizer puts out more than 3 trillion ions per second, regulates itself according to the level of ions in the room, is light and compact, and can easily be moved from office to home or from one room to another.

The Sinus Survival Spray is a botanical nasal spray that contains normal saline (salt water), aloe vera, goldenseal, selenium, and grapefruit seed extract (see p. 153). It not only serves as an irrigant and moisturizer, but its herbal ingredients can help to heal the mucous membrane, diminish allergy symptoms, and lessen the amount of bacteria, viruses, and candida in the nose and sinuses. It is safe and can be used several times daily, both preventively and during allergy seasons and bouts of sinusitis.

The Sinus Survival Cough Drops and Cough Syrup are exciting new herbal products containing echinacea, among other herbs.

Sinus Survival Grape Seed Extract and Sinus Survival Ester C are also available.

The Steam Inhaler is a device I've been using and recommending to patients for the past two years. It's excellent for moistening mucous membranes and helping the sinuses to drain. I recommend that it be used before nasal irrigation, when you feel increased head and nasal congestion, and when you've been exposed to a lot of dirty and/or dry air. Adding a couple of drops of eucalyptus oil to the water is very soothing to the mucous membrane.

If you're interested in additional information or in ordering these products, please refer to the "Product Index" at the end of the book.

6. Should I have sinus surgery?

Although I would need to do a thorough evaluation of your history before rendering a definitive opinion, the answer to this question is usually no. Sinus surgery should always be considered a last resort, when all else has failed. But for most physicians, "all else" usually consists of multiple courses of antibiotics. Physicians who prescribe antibiotics and then offer the option of surgery are almost always otolaryngologists—ear, nose, and throat surgeons. The focus of their training, what they do best and most enjoy doing, and what they are richly rewarded for, is performing surgery. Is it any wonder that the majority of sinus surgeries are unnecessary? Almost $5 billion will be spent this year in the

United States on sinus surgery. If it cured sinus disease it would certainly be worthwhile, but in most cases it does not. This is because the surgical procedure often treats the symptoms rather than the causes of chronic sinusitis.

If your sinuses are filled with polyps or cysts that are blocking the ostia, then I would recommend surgery. To prevent them from recurring, I'd suggest starting the Sinus Survival Program following the surgery. The reason most often given to justify nasal/sinus surgery is a deviated nasal septum, the "dividing wall" between the two nostrils. The majority of people in our society have a deviated septum to some degree, but most of them do not have sinus problems. It is important to realize that if you do have a deviated septum it has been deviated most of your life; but most likely you've had sinus infections only in recent years. The septum is therefore *not* the cause of your problem. It is the swollen mucous membranes covering the septum and the other sides of your nostrils (the turbinates) that are responsible for preventing your sinuses from draining. I'd temporarily forgo surgery and diligently follow the program, especially chapters 8 and 9 along with the "Moisture and Irrigation" section in Chapter 5. If after doing this your condition is unchanged (which is highly unlikely), you can then choose the surgical option, knowing that you've "given it your best shot."

7. Do I need to take antibiotics for every sinus infection?
No. Sinus infections can be treated effectively without antibiotics, if you strictly adhere to the Sinus Survival Program. I would especially recommend steaming followed by irrigation three or four times a day, more sleep, the vitamin and herbal regimen (a natural "antibiotic") prescribed in Chapter 8, and addressing the emotional causes of your infection. It may take about two weeks to feel 100 percent normal and have consistently clear or white mucus. Recovery time will be much shorter if you can identify and treat all of the causes of the sinus infection, especially releasing your anger.

For most of the patients whom I've treated for chronic sinusitis, repeated use of antibiotics has been a primary *cause* of their sinus disease (see p. 60). While weakening their immune system, antibiotics can also lead to an overgrowth of Candida, which can both directly and indirectly worsen their sinuses. If you're someone with type 1 or 2 chronic sinusitis, taking three or more courses of antibiotics within a six-month period, then I would avoid any additional antibiotics in treating your sinus infection. If you have one or two infections per year, then it's probably okay to take an antibiotic; but there's no assurance that it will work any faster than the natural regimen I prescribe in this book. If your experience has you convinced that you can get better only by taking the drug, then take the antibiotic along with acidophilus, in addition to steaming, irrigation, sleep, and the vitamin/ herbal regimen. If you're someone who's had candidiasis in the past and you now have a sinus infection, I'd be suspicious of Candida as a factor contributing to this infection. In this case, add the recommendations from Chapter 9 to your treatment of the sinus infection.

8. What vitamin dosages and diet modifications do you recommend for children and for pregnant women?
See the charts at the end of Chapter 8.

9. Does irrigation help only temporarily?
No. Nasal irrigation can potentially be the most therapeutic measure in completely eliminating a sinus infection (see p. 71). It can help quickly and dramatically. I've heard from people who have had an infection for months that within two days of beginning irrigation, the infection was gone and did not return, even if irrigation was not continued beyond a few days.

If the problem is chronic sinusitis, your mucous membranes may have been inflamed and irritated for years, with the cilia badly damaged. In this case, daily irrigation is an essential part of the program used to heal the membranes and prevent further infection. The bathing of the membranes with salt water keeps them moist and eliminates pollutants and particles usually removed by the cilia. While irrigation in this instance helps temporarily (just while you're doing it), it also has the long-term benefit of helping the membranes return to normal.

10. Can I use a combination of conventional and holistic remedies?
Absolutely. In the answer to question 7 I've explained how and when to use antibiotics in conjunction with my holistic Sinus Survival Program. Holistic medicine advocates the use of any safe, gentle, and effective therapy while treating the whole person. It is inclusive of conventional medicine and is best thought of as *complementary,* rather than alternative or unconventional, medicine. Although most conventional medical treatments (surgery and pharmaceutical drugs) are either invasive or are accompanied by unpleasant side effects, there are instances where conventional medicine is preferable. If after considering the pros and cons of all the available options you decide to use a conventional treatment, there are usually holistic measures you can take to minimize the harmful side effects. Vitamins, herbs, steam, irrigation, affirmations, visualization, acupuncture, journaling, and prayer can be quite helpful both before and after sinus surgery. Taking acidophilus along with antibiotics can help to minimize candida overgrowth.

By the end of this decade there will no longer be a clear distinction between conventional and holistic medicine. The cost-effectiveness and therapeutic value of many holistic treatments, including the Sinus Survival Program, are currently being scientifically proven and will soon be incorporated into a greatly expanded list of conventional medical treatment options. I also believe that by the turn of the century holistic medicine will be recognized as conventional medicine's newest specialty.

Chapter 16

CREATING HEALTHY SINUSES AND A HEALTHY LIFE

Having read this far in the book, you know now that the treatment of chronic respiratory disease can encompass the entire spectrum of medicine—from simply taking antibiotics and bronchodilators to engaging in a process that might transform your life. If you choose, this transformation can help you make the transition from dependence on the medical profession and medication, to the recognition that you are capable of healing yourself. A human being, in fact, is an intrinsically self-healing organism, but we have developed many unhealthy habits that make it much more difficult for us to enjoy our lives fully.

In *Sinus Survival* I have shared with you my approach to health, derived from a healing odyssey that began with my roots in conventional allopathic medicine as the son of a radiologist, and that continued through the transitional stage of osteopathic medicine to my current work in what I believe will become the foundation of the health care system of the future: holistic medicine. What began as a desire to improve the condition of my sinuses has led me to a different style of medical practice, a cure for sinus disease and potentially any other chronic condition, and the recognition of a degree of personal health I had never imagined possible.

The only new aspect of this approach is that medical science is now, very slowly, giving it a stamp of approval through the fields

321

of nutrition, environmental medicine, behavioral medicine, and psychoneuroimmunology. Many so-called primitive cultures, much less technologically developed than our own, have instinctively practiced variations of holistic medicine. In the developed world holistic medicine is a comprehensive approach that incorporates everything from ancient healing practices to space-age technologies.

As a family doctor, I spent most of the past twenty-three years trying to find simple, quick, painless, and effortless remedies to satisfy my patients' requests for fast relief of their discomfort. During the past eight years as a holistic physician, however, I've learned that a desire for the "quick fix" is one of the greatest obstacles to health. The need to immediately relieve physical discomfort has spawned a pharmaceutical industry that has responded with a drug for almost every symptom, but has not prepared us for the serious consequences of adverse side effects and drug dependence. The approach I offer in this book synthesizes my family practice orientation as a "fixer" of symptoms, friend, and counselor (time permitting) with the focus of holistic medicine—the physician serving as a facilitator and coach in the patient's self-healing "training program."

If you are willing to make the commitment to the Sinus Survival Program, you will be giving yourself life's greatest gift—health. Far beyond the mere relief of sinus headaches, a stuffy nose, sneezing, or wheezing, *optimal health is a feeling of being much more alive.* Its primary expense seems to be our society's most precious commodity: time. If you are not in a hurry, you've got it made, and you might be surprised to find that the program doesn't take nearly as much time out of your daily schedule as you thought it would. Many of the methods and practices I have described require only a heightened awareness on your part and very little extra time. However, you do need to slow down to develop greater sensitivity to the needs of your body, mind, and spirit.

Just as with any training program, you must be willing to practice before you can attain a new level of fitness. You need to set goals that are within your reach. Think of it as a process of taking "baby steps." But remember that even before a toddler is ready for those first steps, he or she must first learn to crawl, then stand, followed by a series of failed attempts at walking. Yet there's always progress, since there's something to be learned with each fall.

The initial goal for almost everyone who begins the Sinus Survival Program is to either relieve symptoms, avoid surgery, or stop taking antibiotics, antihistamines, inhalers, cortisone tablets and sprays, or allergy shots. That's why I recommended at the beginning of the book that you start the program by working on *physical* and *environmental* health as described in chapters 7 and 8, and prepare a symptom chart (see pp. 129–30) that also includes the medications and dosages that you will be taking as you start. If you are already taking an antibiotic or have been on a long-term (more than two to three months) nasal steroid spray, then I would stop them both. The asthma inhalers and cortisone tablets have to be tapered very gradually, as I've previously described. With asthma, it's best initially to work with your physician in tapering your medications.

I realize that there is quite a bit to do and many changes to make during this first phase, so implement the steps at a pace that feels comfortable and affordable to you. Try to practice and implement as many of the physical and environmental recommendations as you can for a full month, before adding mental health to the training regimen. Exercise is the part of the physical program that's most often neglected, takes the most time, and seems to be the most difficult to initiate. I'd suggest that you very gradually work up to the lower limit of your fitness heart rate (take the entire month to get up to this level and maintain it for only ten minutes or less, three times a week). Regular exercise might eventually pay the greatest dividends of any aspect of the entire program. For those of you who were already engaged in an aerobic exercise program, I'd suggest cutting back on your workouts and making it very easy on yourself (and your immune system) during these first four weeks.

If you experience only minimal symptom improvement after the first month, I would then incorporate the treatment of candida into your program for the second month (especially if you have been on long-term antibiotics and/or cortisone), before starting to work on your psychological well-being.

By the time you're ready to begin practicing *mental* health, you will have either experienced a marked improvement in your symptoms, postponed surgery, been off antibiotics for one month, or reduced your dosage of cortisone and inhalers. In any case, you will have taken a rather large step from where you had been a month or two earlier, one that you might not have believed possible just a short time ago. Not only does your body feel better, you're also experiencing greater self-esteem—proud of yourself for having taken this risk and been rewarded for it. You're also changing a limiting belief, or several of them, in the process, e.g., "Well, maybe I don't have to live with this ____ [sinusitis, asthma, etc.] after all." You are already mentally healthier before even beginning this second stage of the program.

The single most helpful exercise in the mental health aspect of the program is the goal list. This is your personal vision and becomes your blueprint for restructuring your life. As you reinforce this new direction on a daily basis by reciting, writing, and/or visualizing your affirmations, you will develop a greater sense of well-being. Most of my patients report that the recitation of their affirmations always makes them feel better. Although it might take several hours or even days initially to formulate your goal list and reword it into affirmations, the exercise itself could take from five to twenty minutes a day, depending upon the length of your list. In the course of just one month of daily practice you will be surprised to see how many of your goals are at least partially realized, and how much more easily you can recognize your limiting beliefs and hear the self-critical messages you give yourself. Practicing forgiveness is an integral part of holistic health. The affirmation "I am always doing the best I can" is a valuable addition to almost anyone's list.

Now that you're "on a roll," you should be ready to handle *emotional* health. The primary objective of this phase of your training is to learn to feel all of your feelings. You can begin to accomplish this just by identifying it as one of the goals on your list. Anger release, meditation, and play are the three emotional health techniques that are most helpful to incorporate initially.

For most of my patients, some form of anger release on a daily basis has been immediately beneficial. This can take only a minute or less to do. I realize it feels awkward at first, but that's because venting anger seems so unnatural. Keep in mind that had it been more natural for us to express our anger when we were younger, such "training" wouldn't be necessary.

Meditation serves as a highly effective means of identifying your feelings. Begin with at least five to ten minutes a day—and don't worry about "doing it right." Remember there are no mistakes, only lessons.

And don't forget to play. If you regularly participate in a sport or a moderately strenuous physical activity, you're fulfilling your emotional need to "get out of your head and into your body," i.e., to play. If you don't, choose something that's relaxing, creative, or just plain fun—and give yourself at least an hour each week to enjoy it.

Depending upon your degree of commitment to the Sinus Survival Program, after three or four months you will probably be feeling much better. In fact, according to a recent survey I conducted on all of my chronic sinusitis patients in the past six years, 92 percent of those who had strictly adhered to the program for at least the first two full months now consider their sinusitis to be either cured (no infections and no sinus symptoms) or of the type 3 variety (only one or two infections per year, with minimal or no chronic symptoms). Almost all of these people had been either type 1 or 2 (either continual infection or three or more infections within a six-month period) when they began the program.

At this stage, your awareness of your body—what makes it feel better or worse—will be much greater than it has ever been. The longer the duration of your infection-, allergy-, or asthma-free periods, the more sensitive you'll become to the earliest symptom of physical dysfunction. The sooner you respond to your body's warning signs, the more effectively you will be able to prevent sinus infections and allergy and asthma attacks.

The other important lesson you'll learn at this stage is that you've become much more conscious of your feelings, critical self-talk, and the way in which your attitudes affect your sense of well-being. If you have any "setbacks" (sinus infections, allergy or asthma attacks) during these first few months, which is often the case, then you'll be given an excellent opportunity to learn more about the inextricably bound mind-body connection. Whenever an infection occurs, pay attention to what you were thinking and feeling and what was going on in your life in the twenty-four to forty-eight hours preceding its onset. Rather than representing a regression or failure because you "got another one of these damn sinus infections," these illnesses allow you to deepen your practice of the Sinus Survival training.

It will take time for your immune system to be restored to its full capacity. So expect a continued vulnerability to infection, allergy, and asthma for several months. After two or three months of Sinus Survival practice, you'll be able to observe more easily how painful feelings or persistent critical beliefs can make you sick.

And as you become more in tune with your emotional, mental, and spiritual needs, you'll begin to see how this incredible self-healing organism—your body—is continuously acting as your guide. It is teaching you how to care for it not only with good food, enough water, and exercise, but with more nurturing thoughts and feelings as well. The better you understand this process, the more exciting and life-giving it becomes. The one-year-old who continues to fall in his attempts to walk doesn't get discouraged and think, "I'll never be able to walk." Instead, he becomes more animated and thrilled with his progress as he gets up to try again. Knowing that you are not alone on this healing path, and that there is a great deal of help (actually an infinite supply) out there (and in there) for you is the greatest benefit of *spiritual* health.

This is a challenging training program. To make the commitment to transform your life is a risk that few people are willing to take. Why? Because change is scary, and the fear of the unknown presents too formidable an obstacle for most of us to overcome.

Thomas Jefferson wrote in the Declaration of Independence that people would rather suffer than change. Basic human nature is no different today than it was more than 200 years ago. There is a comfort or familiarity in being miserable with the known, rather than subjecting oneself to the insecurity of the unknown.

Although it may not be as clearly defined as something you can experience with your five senses, you are given clear feedback regarding your spiritual health on a regular basis. The information comes to you not through your mind or intellect but is transmitted through your heart—your connection to spirit. The more you practice learning to listen, the better you will be able to receive the nurturing and caring messages that flow through this direct conduit to unconditional love. As you commit to a minimal amount of time on a daily and weekly basis for your spiritual training—prayer or meditation, gratitude, spiritual practices, Sabbath, touch—you will hear your intuition, or the voice of God, speaking to you much more clearly. He or She speaks the language of love. The more you learn to trust and act upon this compassionate inner voice, the less fear you will have and the easier it will be for you to strengthen your commitment to change and to heal.

In the final stage of your basic training program, you are now prepared to apply to your "neighbor"—spouse, partner, children —what you've been practicing on yourself. *Social* health can potentially be a powerful demonstration of your degree of spiritual growth. Creating intimate relationships has been the most challenging aspect of the Sinus Survival Program for the majority of my patients, and the lack of intimacy, one of the primary causes of chronic dis-ease. Much of the anger that ignites sinus infections is often directed at spouses and partners. If you are in a marriage or a committed relationship and your partner is willing, I would suggest starting with the listening exercise at least once a week. The benefits are immediate, as it diminishes the almost universal fear of intimacy. If you are single and not in a committed relationship, you may have a close friend with whom you'd like to practice this communication exercise.

The Sinus Survival Program has the potential to transform

your life. Eliminating sinus and respiratory disease is only the beginning. At least six months of committing to loving yourself in body (environmental and physical health), mind (mental and emotional health), and spirit (spiritual and social health) is the minimum amount of time for this transformation to occur. It depends on your level of commitment and how much you're willing to practice. With sufficient dedication to your own well-being, you will develop healthy habits that will allow you to maintain and improve upon your holistic health. You will acquire the skills to heal yourself and be much more in control of how you feel on a day-to-day basis. As long as you continue to learn from occasional episodes of illness, you will continue to take your Sinus Survival training program to higher levels.

The image I have of this process is of a dynamic upright spiral, like a gigantic metal spring standing on end, with the bottom rung firmly entrenched in the earth and the upper end ascending out of sight. Every level of the spring consists of body, mind, and spirit, held in perfect balance. As you deepen your level of self-awareness in each aspect of your life, you find yourself moving upward along the spiral and enjoying a greater degree of health. The speed of this process is different for each of us—our choices control the accelerator. The most powerful impetus for most of us to leave the security and comfort of our present plateau in life and move on to the next higher level is crisis—a physical, emotional, or spiritual crisis. The Chinese symbol for crisis has two meanings—danger and opportunity.

Holistic health requires time—there is no quick fix. To change your behavior and re-create your life requires a commitment to yourself that will probably be greater than any you've ever made. So too will be the rewards. In your willingness to take this risk, you will be embarking on a healing journey that I hope you'll continue for the rest of your life. This book will help you to get started, but you should be able to navigate quite well on your own the rest of the way.

Each of you has your own benevolent inner healer who is eminently more qualified to work with you and knows you far better than I. He or She is with you every moment of every day.

You can have daily private consultations that cost far less than mine would. Don't be surprised if at times the guidance you receive sounds like it's coming from your inner child, and that this process of re-creation feels a lot like recreation. Holistic health means living life to its fullest. As you follow the program in Part II of this book, many of you will progress from a state of survival to one of thriving. It is a true life-changing adventure. Have fun! I'll be with you in spirit.

PRODUCT INDEX

—Adrenal Complex: available only to health care practitioners through DS Vitamins, 1-800-435-2699.

—Bionaire Climate Check (measures temperature and humidity): available in some hardware and department stores; call 1-800-253-2764 (in U.S.) or 1-800-561-6478 (in Canada) to find the store nearest you.

—Bionaire Clear Mist 5 (CMP-5), tabletop humidifier: available in many hardware and some department stores; call 1-800-253-2764 (in U.S.) or 1-800-561-6478 (in Canada) to find the store nearest you.

—Clear Tox (for leaky gut syndrome): available in some health food stores or through Klabin Marketing at 1-800-933-9440.

—Columbus Industries' furnace filter called "The Magnet" (Magnet High Efficiency Allergy Relief Filter): available at Sears and some hardware and mass merchandisers; or call 1-800-288-8955.

—Dupont Hysurf vacuum cleaner bags: available in some janitorial supply houses and medical supply stores or through Healthy Habitats at (303) 671-9653.

—Dupont Wizard dustcloth: available in some janitorial supply houses or through Healthy Habitats at (303) 671-9653.

—Flora Balance (bacteria for treating candida): available in many health food stores or through Bio-Nutritional Formulas at 1-800-950-8484.

—Grossan Nasal Irrigator: available in some pharmacies or through Hydromed, Inc., at 1-800-560-9007.

—Intestinalis (herbal combination for treating candida): available in some health food stores or through Bio-Nutritional Formulas at 1-800-950-8484.

—Kenmore Warm Mist, tabletop humidifier: available at most Sears stores.

—Mycocan Combo (homeopathic for treating candida): available only to health care practitioners through Mountain States Health Care Products at 1-800-647-0074.

—Neti Pot (for nasal irrigation): available in some health food stores or through the Himalayan Institute at 1-800-822-4547.

—Proanthocyanidin (grape seed extract, or pycnogenol): available in some health food stores, or as Sinus Survival Grape Seed Extract through Klabin Marketing at 1-800-933-9440.

—Rhinotherm unit: available through Netzer Integrated Technologies; North American sales manager at (303) 466-0797, or Creative Distribution Services at (201) 926-5606.

—Room Air Cleaners:

1. Air Purifier/Ion generator combinations: available in many hardware and department stores, or for Bionaire F-150 or F-250 call Bionaire numbers previously mentioned.
2. HEPA Air Cleaners: available in many hardware and department stores.
3. Negative Ion Generators: available in some hardware and department stores, or for Sinus Survival Air Vitalizer through Air Tech International at (303) 530-3934.

—Sinus Survival Candidetect: pending FDA approval, this test will probably be available sometime in 1996 through Klabin Marketing at 1-800-933-9440.

—Sinus Survival Cough Drops and Cough Syrup; available in some health food stores or through Klabin Marketing at 1-800-933-9440.

—Sinus Survival Spray: available in some health food stores or through Klabin Marketing at 1-800-933-9440.

—Steam Inhaler: available in some pharmacies or through Bernhard Industries at 1-800-544-6425.

—Test Kit for Indoor Allergens (mold, dust mite, cat, roach): available through Healthy Habitats at (303) 671-9653.

—Ultra Clear: available only to health care practitioners through Metagenics at 1-800-692-9400.

—V-VAX Eucalyptus oil: available in some health food stores or through V-VAX Products at (312) 276-1747.

—Vitamin C, as an ascorbate or as Ester C: available in most health food stores or as Sinus Survival Ester C through Klabin Marketing at 1-800-933-9440.

BIBLIOGRAPHY

Adinoff, Allen D. "Difficult Asthma? Look for Sinusitis." *National Jewish Center for Immunology and Respiratory Medicine Medical Scientific Update,* February 1987.

Anderson, Robert A. *Wellness Medicine.* New Canaan, Conn.: Keats, 1990.

Anand, Margo. *The Art of Sexual Ecstasy.* Los Angeles: J. P. Tarcher, 1989.

Bandler, Richard. *Using Your Brain for a Change.* Moab, Utah: Real People Press, 1985.

Bauer, Cathryn. *Acupressure for Everybody.* New York: Henry Holt, 1991.

Benedict, Martha S. "Holistic Approaches to Colds and Flu." *Body Mind Spirit,* February/March 1995.

Byrd, Randolph C. "Positive Therapeutic Effects of Intercessory Prayer in a Coronary Care Unit Population." *Southern Medical Journal,* July 1988.

Carey, Benedict. "A Jog in the Smog." *Hippocrates,* May/June 1989.

Carper, Jean. *Food—Your Miracle Medicine.*

Challem, Jack. "Defend Yourself Against Supergerms." *Natural Health,* March/April 1995.

Cherry, Rona. "The Best News of the Year." *Longevity,* May 1991.

Clerico, Dean M., and David W. Kennedy. "Chronic Sinusitis: Diagnostic and Treatment Advances." *Hospital Medicine,* July 1994.

Cooper, Robert K. *Health and Fitness Excellence.* New York: Houghton Mifflin, 1989.

Cotton, Paul. " 'Best Data Yet' Say Air Pollution Kills Below Levels

Currently Considered Safe." *Journal of the American Medical Association,* June 23/30, 1993.

Crerand, Joanne. "Home Remedy: Insomnia." *Natural Health,* March/April 1992.

Crowther, Richard L. *Indoor Air: Risks and Remedies.* Denver: Directions Publishing, 1989.

Dockery, Douglas W., C. Arden Pope III, Xiphing Xu, John D. Spengler, James H. Ware, Martha E. Fay, Benjamin G. Ferris, Jr., and Frank E. Speizer. "An Association Between Air Pollution and Mortality in Six U.S. Cities." *The New England Journal of Medicine,* December 9, 1993.

Dossey, Larry. *Healing Words.* San Francisco: Harper, 1993.

Dreher, Henry. "Why Did the People of Roseto Live So Long?" *Natural Health,* September/October 1993.

Feltman, John, ed. *Hands-on Healing: Massage Remedies for Hundreds of Health Problems.* Emmaus, Penn.: Rodale Press, 1989.

Firshein, Richard. "Treating Asthma Without Drugs." *Natural Health,* July/August 1994.

Gaby, Alan R. "Human Canaries and Silent Spring." *Holistic Medicine: Magazine of the American Holistic Medical Association,* Fall/Winter 1992.

Gantz, Nelson M., Donald Kaye, C. Wayne Weart. "Antibiotics '95: Back to Basics." *Patient Care,* January 15, 1995.

Gray, Henry. *Anatomy of the Human Body.* 8th ed., Charles Mayo Goss, ed. Philadelphia: Lea and Febiger, 1967.

Growald, Eileen Rockefeller, and Allan Luks. "The Healing Power of Doing Good." *American Health,* March 1988.

Guyton, Arthur C. *Textbook of Medical Physiology.* Philadelphia: W. B. Saunders Company, 1968.

Hay, Louise L. *You Can Heal Your Life.* Santa Monica, Calif.: Hay House, 1984.

Hendeles, Leslie, Miles Weinberger, and Lai Wong. "Medical Management of Noninfectious Rhinitis." *American Journal of Hospital Pharmacy,* November 1980.

Hendrix, Harville. *Getting the Love You Want: A Guide for Couples.* New York: Harper & Row, 1988.

Hersch, Patricia. "The Resounding Silence." *The Family Therapy Networker,* July/August 1990.

Josephson, Jordan S., Seth I. Rosenberg. "Sinusitis." *Clinical Symposia, Ciba,* 1994.

Joy, W. Brugh. *Joy's Way: A Map for the Transformational Journey*. Los Angeles: J. P. Tarcher, 1979.

Kozora, E. J. *American Holistic Medical Association's Nutritional Guidelines*. Seattle: American Holistic Medical Association, 1987.

Krakovitz, Rob. *High Energy: How to Overcome Fatigue and Maintain Your Peak Vitality*. New York: Ballantine Books, 1986.

Langs, Robert. "Understanding Your Dreams." *New Age Journal*, July/August 1988.

LaPerriere, Arthur, Gail Ironson, Michael H. Antoni, Neil Schneiderman, Nancy Klimas, and Mary Ann Fletcher. "Exercise and Psychoneuroimmunology." *American College of Sports Medicine,* 1994.

Maharishi Ayur-Veda Newsletter. "Sleep Like a Baby: The Ayurvedic Approach to Insomnia." September 1992.

National Institute of Allergy and Infectious Diseases. "Sinusitis." Bethesda, Maryland, 1989.

Neile, Caren. "Banish Allergies Forever!" Globe Communications Corp., 1991.

Ophir, Dov, and Yigal Elad. "Effects of Steam Inhalation on Nasal Patency and Nasal Symptoms in Patients with the Common Cold." *American Journal of Otolaryngology,* 1987.

Ophir, Dov, Yigal Elad, Zvi Dolev, and Carmi Geller-Bernstein. "Effects of Inhaled Humidified Warm Air on Nasal Patency and Nasal Symptoms in Allergy Rhinitis." *Annals of Allergy,* March 1988.

Ornstein, Robert, and David Sobel. *Healthy Pleasures*. New York: Addison-Wesley, 1989.

Parker, Sharon. "Drugs vs. the Bug." *Utne Reader,* March/April 1995.

Patent, Arnold. *You Can Have It All*. Great Neck, N.Y.: Money Mastery, 1984.

Peck, M. Scott. *The Road Less Traveled*. New York: Simon and Schuster, 1978.

Rapp, Doris. *Allergies and Your Family*. Buffalo, N.Y.: Practical Allergy, 1990.

Reid, Clyde. *Celebrate the Temporary*. New York: Harper & Row, 1972.

Ruddy, John R. "Diagnosing and Treating Sleep Disorders." *National Jewish Center for Immunology and Respiratory Medicine Medical/Scientific Update,* April 1993.

Scarf, Maggie. *Intimate Partners*. New York: Random House, 1987.

Siegel, Bernie S. *Love, Medicine and Miracles*. New York: Harper and Row, 1986.

South Coast Air Quality Management District. *Where Does It Hurt?:*

Bibliography

Answers to Questions about Smog and Health. El Monte, California, 1988.

Spangler, Tina. "The Solution for Indoor Pollution." *Natural Health,* January/February 1995.

Togias, Alkis G. et al. Robert M. Nacierio, David Proud. "Nasal Challenge with Dry Cold Air in Release of Inflammatory Mediators: Possible Mast Cell Involvement." The American Society for Clinical Investigation, October 1985.

United States Department of Health and Human Services, Public Health Service, National Institutes of Health, National Asthma Education Program. "Executive Summary: Guidelines for the Diagnosis and Management of Asthma," June 1991.

United States Environmental Protection Agency, Office of Air Quality Planning and Standards Technical Support Division. *National Air Quality and Emissions Trend Report,* 1993. Research Triangle Park, North Carolina, 1994.

Vital and Health Statistics, from the Centers for Disease Control and Prevention/National Center for Health Statistics. "Current Estimates From the National Health Interview Survey," 1992.

Warga, Claire. "You Are What You Think." *Psychology Today,* September 1988.

Yerushalmi, Aharon, Sergiu Karman, and Andre Lwoff. "Treatment of perennial allergic rhinitis by local hyperthermia." Proc. *National Academy of Science USA,* August 1982.

INDEX

Index

Index

Index

Index

Index

About the Author

Robert Ivker completed his medical training in 1972 in his hometown, at the Philadelphia College of Osteopathic Medicine. In 1975, following a family medicine residency at Mercy Medical Center in Denver, Colorado, he opened a solo practice just outside the Mile-High City. The practice flourished, and in 1983 he established Columbine Medical Center, consisting of five family doctors. Today there is a network of several Columbine Centers based on his prototype, making up the largest family practice in the state. These facilities are all owned and operated by Porter Memorial Hospital.

Since leaving Columbine in 1987, he has devoted his career to writing —this is the third edition of *Sinus Survival,* and his next book, *Thriving: A Man's Guide to Creating Optimal Health and Fitness,* will be published in 1997—and to practicing holistic medicine. This practice is focused on treating chronic disease and teaching patients how to create holistic health, while strengthening his commitment to do the same thing for himself.

Dr. Ivker has been board-certified by the American Board of Family Practice, is a Fellow of the American Academy of Family Physicians, and is a member of the board of trustees of the American Holistic Medical Association; he will become president of that organization in 1996. He is a clinical instructor in the Departments of Otolaryngology and Family Medicine at the University of Colorado School of Medicine.

Married for twenty-seven years to Harriet, a clinical social worker specializing in marriage and family therapy, he and his wife live in Littleton, Colorado, with their daughters Julie and Carin.